D0591218

14-120-1279

DEVELOPING
THE SUPERVISORY SKILLS
OF THE NURSE:

A BEHAVIORAL SCIENCE APPROACH

DEVELOPING
THE SUPERVISORY SKILLS
OF THE NURSE

A BEHAVIORAL SCIENCE APPROACH

ADELMA E. MOOTH, ED.D., R.N., Professor of Nursing, and Chairman of Programs in Nursing Service Administration, School of Nursing, Boston University

MIRIAM M. RITVO, B.A., M.S., Training Associate, Human Relations Center, Boston University; Assistant Professor, School of Education, Boston University; and Lecturer, School of Nursing, Boston University

The Macmillan Company, New York
Collier-Macmillan Limited, London

First Printing

Library of Congress catalog card number: 66-14210

THE MACMILLAN COMPANY, NEW YORK
COLLIER-MACMILLAN CANADA, LTD.,
TORONTO, ONTARIO

PRINTED IN THE UNITED STATES OF AMERICA

. . . When you assemble a number of men to have the advantage of their joint wisdom you inevitably assemble with those men all their prejudices, their passions, their errors of opinion, their local interests, and their selfish views. It therefore astonishes me, Sir, to find this system approaching so near to perfection as it does.

Benjamin Franklin

To all the participants who have been co-learners with us in the seminars, training laboratories, and in-service programs we have conducted over the years in hospitals, educational institutions, and industry. You have made our behavioral science theories come alive.

In all the particulars which have been under review, as in the seminate mating temperature and in-vivo processes, we have considered two devices to begin with—the classical distinction, and indeed — — — — — — released within the si— was — — — — —

PREFACE

The purpose of this book is to serve the special and growing need for improved in-service supervisory programs in hospitals. We want to call attention to the often neglected fact that in-service education *is* adult education. Our philosophy of supervision in nursing is based on behavioral science concepts that are consistent with and complementary to theories of adult education. Participative, collaborative supervision as a process has the same theoretical and practical base that we find in the adult education world.

Many research studies in both the fields of organizational behavior and the adult learner increasingly support the assumptions that the supervised and the adult learner are more effective and involved when they participate in the process; if they are consulted about decisions that will affect them; if a climate of trust exists between levels; if there is a two-way instead of a "tell 'em" communication pattern; if shared, not imposed, goals are the norm. Laboratory and field studies conducted by behavioral scientists demonstrate that the behavior and attitudes of the immediate supervisor affect the subordinate's performance in an almost predictable manner. We champion the twin theories that supportive, participative supervision and adult teacher-learner partnership elicit the highest productivity and morale.

The concrete reality about most in-service programs is that administration wishes to influence behavior toward the achievement of organizational goals and at the same time wants to increase individual job satisfaction. If these goals are equally valid, the use of the appropriate in-service method is critical. In the rapidly expanding field of adult education, many new methods are used to maximize learning. This book focuses on the case method because it is the one that uses the principles and processes of the educative supervisory style we are describing. Our goal is to fuse the behavioral science implications of supervision with adult education by the use of the case method.

The selected cases and situations contained in this book deal with a range of supervisory situations that actually occurred in a variety of hospital settings. The cases highlight day-to-day problems and processes. They provide a framework for participants to use in the analysis, diagnosis, and action plan for the improvement of a variety of supervisory situations. Each case invites the discussant to consider the definition of the problem, decisions to be made, data needed, weighing of variables, reality-testing possible solutions, testing the relative merits of alternatives, and figuring the results and risks in any decision. As we see it, all these processes involve working with and through people, so a focus of analysis must be the human, the "people" side of supervision. Each case should be used to examine the behavioral aspects implicit in every supervisory function.

We see nursing supervision as a process, not just a position or category; it occurs at all levels. Since *levels are people*—adults, at that—we hope the case analysis approach will help participants to develop and enhance their supervisory judgments, sensitivity, and understanding.

There is no attempt to provide "answers" or to suggest that solutions can be classified in correct and incorrect categories. Experience tells us many supervisory situations involve such a complex of factors that it would be unrealistic and "gimmicky" to search for *the* answer. Our goal is to provide the opportunity through the study and discussion of these cases for participants to develop a more mature, dynamic, and human way of looking at each problem. Stated another way, the training emphasis is on the process of coping, not the mechanics, though both coexist and interact.

We hope that each participant in this in-service program will grow objective enough to see that her own behavior and attitudes are always part of the situation and therefore influence the way she typically handles people and problems. In dealing with the behavioral processes which are often the core of a situation, we hope that the discussant will examine the role of *self*.

In this book, we have tried something new in the use of the case method. Usually, an experienced, outside person is selected to do the teaching. We believe that it is possible for a hospital to "grow" its own case discussion leader. For this purpose, we have included a description of the case method and a detailed guideline section to develop the skills and attitudes for an effective leader-teacher-supervisor. The supervision and adult education sections are self-contained so they may be the basis for discussion even if the cases are not used in the in-service program.

We gratefully acknowledge the assistance of Tuckerman Day, Editorial Consultant, during the writing of the manuscript. To the Boston University Board of Trustees go our special thanks for permission to reprint the copyrighted cases. We wish to thank Mrs. Winifred Griffin, R.N., Associate Director for Regional Nursing Programs, New England Board of Higher Education, and Nurse Consultant to the New England Council on Higher Education for Nursing, for granting the use of modified unpublished case materials.

A. E. M.
M. M. R.

CONTENTS

DEVELOPING
THE SUPERVISORY SKILLS
OF THE NURSE:

A BEHAVIORAL SCIENCE APPROACH

1

WHY THIS BOOK?

The historian of a century from now may well describe our era as a time when man learned—or failed to learn—to control the results of his own inventions. This is precisely the situation of the modern hospital, where discoveries and developments carry rich benefits but also present fresh problems.

More specifically, the increasing complexity of patient care and its supervision is making human relations correspondingly intricate and their difficulties baffling; this in turn demands a reshaping of supervisory policies. We have sought to develop a dynamic philosophy of supervision that will be more productive than the traditional system of fixed rules and rigidly standardized procedures. We are interested in helping those responsible for supervising others to increase their skills in observing, diagnosing, and evaluating the complexities encountered in the human problems of hospitals.

This book does not suggest a program for telling supervisors how to behave, or one that prescribes "six steps for problem-solving and four steps for decision-making." Such methods would have been effective in the past, when the hospital was a relatively stable and predictable environment; they cannot cope with the complexities existent in the often turbulent hospital world of today. Paradoxically, increased specialization means increased interdependence among and between departments. This fact makes

1

centralized decision-making at the top inappropriate for attaining organizational and individual goals.

Anyone who supervises the performance of another must recognize how her own and others' attitudes impinge on each interaction and what effects they have on collaborative efforts. Often an attempt to weld a team consists of little more than pooling jobs instead of pooling commitments. There is a need for the supervisor to improve her skills in diagnosing the motivations and actions of others—a development of personal acuity.

To a large extent supervision means decision-making. The attempt to reach solutions often involves a mixture of uncertainty, compromise, reversal of judgment, and consultation with others in a climate of urgency. Too many times organizational restraints and pressures place such a premium on quick and efficient decisions that cooperative resolution of situations is inhibited, with complexities unexamined and undiagnosed.

So much for goals. What about the ways of achieving them? We believe that in-service training via the case method is the best means of improving supervision in the hospital. We shall tell you about this method and what we have learned from its use.

We then present selected cases which will help you to feel intimately the tensions and pressures of the situations concerned. Emphasis is placed on the principles of supervision drawn from the behavioral sciences. The purpose is to help to develop supervisory skills in analyzing a problem, gathering relevant information, inventing and testing alternative solutions, thinking through tentative consequences, and reanalyzing and evaluating for the best line of action. We can increase our competence in resolving conflict situations by problem-solving rather than through punishment or suppression. All the cases are disguised but present actual situations. The situations described here do not illustrate "good" and "bad" practices. They have been selected to highlight the day-to-day supervisory problems. These cases involve issues of the type faced by supervisors in a variety of hospital settings. Each case invites the discussant to consider the definition of the problem, the data needed, supervisory decisions to be made, weighing of variables, planning of action, and assessing the possible consequences.

Suggested questions are appended to each case, but please bear in mind that they are not given as the best or only ones that could be raised. They are designed to focus attention on issues which must be understood if supervision is to be seen in terms of its function and process. Hopefully, these questions will stimulate students to raise a multiplicity of other questions arising from diverse points of view which are coaxed out.

2

THE HOSPITAL SCENE

Every social organization reflects the influences, problems, and tempo of the society that instituted it, and the hospital and its personnel are no exceptions. No hospital is immune to change and a continuing process of adaptation. One has only to read lay and professional literature, or spend some time in a hospital, to understand the problems that have arisen in the field of hospital nursing. The explosion of medical knowledge has brought about unprecedented changes in the care of the patient, and these require complex planning. The physician has handed responsibilities to the nurse that in the past were reserved to him; hospital administration has handed down administrative activities that call for increased skills in planning, coordination, budgeting, and teaching. Complex equipment demands knowledge of scientific principles that were not previously taught to the nurse. The patient population has been receiving better education in the last twenty years, is more mobile, and is more aggressive in demanding the best care the hospital can give.

Because of the demands upon professional nurses for the complex care of the patient, many categories of nonprofessional workers have been introduced. Within the professional nurse category there are the graduates of the diploma program, the associate arts degree program, and the basic collegiate program. All these workers have varying degrees of competency, depending on educational background and intellectual equipment.

It has become increasingly clear that the schools of nursing cannot educate enough nurses to meet the ever-enlarging demand. Therefore, the total personnel of the nursing department (professional as well as nonprofessional) must be utilized to its maximum potential. Personnel to whom certain aspects of care are delegated must be developed on the job, and the professional nurse must be given an opportunity to continue her education there. Since growth and the change it implies should not be accidental, automatic, or capricious, the hospital must assume some responsibility for helping its employees to increase their interpersonal competence in ways that are in keeping with personal and organizational goals. One cannot rely on preemployment training and experience, because of constantly changing needs and arrangements. Nor can reliance be placed on innate competence, because although this sometimes achieves conspicuous success, it is not systematic and cannot always be taught to others who are less gifted.

A Social Structure

The hospital in its social structure is very much like a school system, a factory, or any other large hierarchical organization. Hospitals are staffed by individuals and groups who feel jealousy, hostility, or indifference; their private interests, both conscious and unconscious, may obscure or even negate the primary interests of the institution. Although these persons and groups may not be crippled by interpersonal problems, they are hampered by them. Minor but frustrating encounters may accumulate until they produce massive inner emotional immobility. Gyroscopic self-defense mechanisms may bring about resistance to change in self, to other personalities, to new ideas, to other disciplines, and collectively can deprive the hospital supervisory staff of a healthy atmosphere of fluid interdependence.

Although most of the personnel carrying out the supervisory process are individually well motivated, technically competent, and reasonably sensitive to others' needs, collectively they may present the classic picture of a rigid organizational system. The result may be a conglomeration of separate principalities existing side by side within the hospital, formally acknowledging the power of the same higher authority and sharing the same ultimate goals, but actually carrying on their own specific functions so independently as to be totally unaware of problems in other departments, with which they seem more or less in a state of armed truce. They fail to realize that their interpersonal competence is intertwined with organizational effectiveness in the vital areas of problem-solving, decision-making, and communication within and between departments.

It is not unusual to find that each supervisor, head nurse, charge nurse, and staff nurse has definite views on job requirements and personnel management, which she considers part of herself, part of her special right to belong to the supervisory aristocracy. She jealously guards her little empire against encroachment from above, below, or any side. Rather than viewing each work unit as a state within a nation, she may regard her unit or her professional discipline as a nation in itself. Finally, the goal of technical or professional competence and the goal of meeting human needs are often seen as conflicting—if, indeed, both are recognized.

The primary barriers to attaining these goals lie in personal resistance to change and the consequent change-resistant methods utilized by supervisors in their work. To examine these methods requires exploration of areas which have become so tangled with vines of tradition that some nursing personnel are forced to pass their professional lives in a state of unexamined discomfort, with an unacceptable norm of continued stress and dissatisfaction.

Another obstacle to competent hospital supervision is the prevailing shortage of personnel who have had advanced training in their job specialities. Because of this the staff must be filled in with inexperienced persons or those with less specialized hospital training. Staff members with advanced training are thus compelled to supervise the work of these less-skilled individuals in addition to carrying out their own duties.

Ironically, the reward for excellence in the hospital sphere is promotion *away* from the specialty for which the individual was originally trained to supervisory work in which she has not been trained. In addition, a nurse, for example, who enjoys and excels in bedside nursing may find all her time taken up by administration. The hospital is forced to have increasing amounts of administrative detail handled by persons whose professional training did not stress administration or supervision.

3

SUPERVISION: A DYNAMIC
PROCESS

Look at the organizational chart of your nursing department. You may find a little square box carrying the title "Supervisor." This individual has traditionally been charged with "supervision" of the nursing care carried out on the floors assigned to her. However, if you examine the job description for this individual or analyze her performance, you are likely to find that she is essentially an administrator. Over the years, because of the increasing complexity of the hospital, the supervisor has had delegated to her more and more activities that prevent her from giving leadership in the improvement of patient care. In some cases her contact with floor personnel occupies only a few minutes a day. These persons think of her not as a sustaining member of the team but as an arm of the nursing office.

Just as the supervisor's day is filled with administrative concerns, so is the day of the head nurse. Some head nurses frankly say they are unable to get away from the desk long enough to visit patients, make rounds with doctors, or observe the care being given by their personnel.

Steps are being taken in many hospitals to free these key people for leadership and supervision by employing administrative assistants in the nursing office and unit managers and clerks on the nursing units. But simply relieving head nurses and supervisors of administrative duties is not enough for successful supervision. The situation demands a flexible, dynamic system. Those who carry it out must not only be experts in nursing, but must also understand the underlying principles of human behavior, motivation, and learning. Glance again at the organizational chart. It takes no account of behavioral dynamics or emotional involvement. People in hospitals do not live in squares or move in straight lines. They circulate in an organizational mix composed of patients, doctors, and fellow-workers, who refuse to conform to a strict system of law and order that makes no allowance for emotions and interpersonal reactions.

Whether or not you are aware of it, you, as a supervisor, have a basic philosophy which determines the goals and objectives of your behavior. A philosophy is a system of beliefs that determine attitudes and actions. These beliefs, in turn, arise from your life experiences as a member of a culture and its subgroups—community, neighborhood, family, church, school. Therefore, in order to have guidelines for your performance, you must have some underlying commitments concerning the process of supervision.

Person-Centered Supervision

Supervision is not a position or a job; it is a dynamic process in which the supervising nurse encourages and participates in the development of her subordinates. This kind of supervision is person-centered. It is based on the growing knowledge of causes of human behavior, of human needs, and of motivation.

We believe that supervision constantly changes in method and understanding because of the evolutionary factors present in all supervisory situations. New techniques; changes in social, economic, and ethnic composition of the patient population; varied backgrounds of personnel—all demand flexibility in scope, method, and timing of supervision. Dynamic supervision assumes respect for the individual and her ability, and places a high value on growth potential. It recognizes her right to have a voice in the planning and carrying out of patient care, and in decision-making when implementation of the decision will involve her.

This is not to say that the final decision will please everyone, but each person has had the opportunity to express her views, and to hear an explanation of the rationale underlying the decision. During the consultation process preceding decision-making, the administrator, supervisor, and head nurse have a wonderful opportunity to teach, to interpret, and to motivate the worker. Situations in all health agencies are so complex today that those removed from the arena of specific problems cannot know all the details; therefore, decisions made with the help of those at the grass roots are likely to be more realistic than those made by the leaders at the top.

In order to participate fruitfully in decision-making and planning, individuals must be aware of the planning that is going on in other groups, so that there can be coordination and a minimum of conflict; in this way supervision "by crisis" can be reduced. When there is ongoing collaboration, problems can be anticipated. The one who is carrying out the supervisory process must develop skill in communication in order to utilize all channels and methods for accomplishing this.

Key Elements in Supervision

There is convincing research evidence that problems arising in supervision can best be solved through the scientific approach and by involving those most affected by the consequences of decision-making.

Dynamic supervision recognizes the importance of intercommunication and interpretation for effective performance. When the individual being supervised understands her role and place in the organization and is continually involved in what is being planned, she can effectively contribute to group effort and thus gain increased satisfaction in her work.

Acceptance of supervision as a dynamic process and not a position necessarily changes the traditional concept of its function. The increasing complexity of the goals of patient care, and the introduction of categories of personnel with varying capabilities, demand that supervision be done by nurses at all levels. Unless this principle is applied, there will be gaps in the development and maintenance of nursing care standards. The nurse who holds the designated title of supervisor is no longer able to cope with the span of control traditionally delegated to her.

The main purposes of dynamic supervision are necessarily developmental and educative. Nurses at each level must function as agents of change so that nursing patterns will meet the health needs of modern society. Improvements in the performance of nursing personnel are brought about through an ongoing educative process which encourages, motivates, instructs, and fosters collaboration for professional and personal development.

Once the foregoing philosophy has been formulated, it has to be translated into action. There are three key elements in this commitment: improvement, encouragement, and participation. They imply personal involvement in bringing about change in the performance of individuals so that the goals of the patient, worker, and supervisor are brought into harmony. This will result in improved care of the patient, as well as personal and professional satisfaction to the worker and supervisor. The role of the supervisor being predominantly educative, the proper focus is on bringing about change in the overt and covert behavior of the one being taught. It is true that administrative functions are involved in defining the goals for bringing about improvement, planning for the change, and evaluating the results of the planning. However, the administrative functions are not the primary ones; they are aids in accomplishing the primary educative goals.

To encourage and participate in the professional and personal development of others requires that one gives of one's self and uses one's self to assist others. It means that one must identify oneself with those caring for the patient and become a member of the ward team. The traditional behavior of the supervisor is incompatible with this commitment. She has functioned as an extended arm of the nursing office and in many cases has been divorced from active participation in the planning and carrying out of patient care. She has been involved primarily in carrying information from the nursing office, collecting reports, sending additional help when needed, hunting for equipment, and doing many other jobs that could be delegated to an administrative assistant, who incidentally need not be a professional person.

Every Nurse a Supervisor

Although it is true that the organizational character of the nursing service imposes on the delegated supervisor activities that prevent her from achieving the primary purpose of supervision, she herself frequently contributes to this situation. The traditional role is less threatening, and she does not have to give so much of herself in performing it. Nevertheless, commitment to the primary purpose of supervision necessarily leads her to find ways to bring about changes in her role.

Furthermore, supervision should not be left entirely to the person carrying the title of supervisor. Responsibility for its execution is inherent in the positions of director of nurses, assistant director, head nurse, assistant head nurse, team leader, and general staff nurse, whether or not they realize this.* As the supervisory process flows down the organizational structure of the nursing service, it becomes more specific in detail and in activity. The head nurse supervises her personnel in giving care. The staff nurses may supervise the aide or student in giving care, or the patient when he gives himself his insulin, or a member of the family who must give the insulin after the discharge of the patient. This downward flow can be illustrated by an inverted triangle, thus:

 DIRECTOR OF NURSES
ASSISTANT DIRECTOR
SUPERVISOR
HEAD NURSE
STAFF NURSE AND TEAM LEADER

Such delegation distributes the burden of responsibility throughout the nursing service and fosters the development of supervisory skills at every level. It becomes the responsibility of the delegated

* In keeping with this concept, the term "supervisor" is used hereafter to designate any individual, at whatever level, who has inherent responsibility for supervision.

supervisor to include in her improvement plans the development of supervisory skills in these individuals at all levels.

Circular Communication

Although supervisory responsibility is delegated in a pyramidal pattern, it extends itself horizontally, involving individuals in all areas of the organization. This sharing of control and responsibility can open channels of communication and cooperation that will change the traditional authority-obedience relationship. It creates a sense of involvement and recognition (ego identification), which releases individuals to contribute to mutual goals; a kind of circular communication is born.

Organizational research findings demonstrate convincingly that sharing relationships dramatically reduce interlevel and intralevel friction. Similarly, tension and discrepancies between individual and organizational goals are lessened. Mutual confidence and trust are the new rewards of collaborative supervision.

The traditional, unilateral supervisory model is static and suppressive and therefore inappropriate for meeting individual and organizational needs. Methods of supervision must go beyond "telling" and into more creative and complex ways of developing people.

The dynamic supervisor must be a student not only of the behavioral components of supervision, but also of the art and science of nursing. This statement may seem tinged with the absurd, but there is plenty of evidence that the supervisor is not expected to be an expert in the field of nursing. She is more often than not perceived as an adjunct to administration and not a clinical specialist. In fact, her self-image may reinforce this perception.

In order to successfully supervise others, the dynamic supervisor must continually investigate the newest literature in her clinical specialty, and the field of nursing in general. She must engage in dialogue with her nursing colleagues, and with members of the health and helping professions. She must take the initiative in building a collaborative relationship with physicians, administrators, and other members of the health team. This is an essential learning experience for her if she is to enlarge her clinical expertise. It is fusion of knowledge of the human side of supervision with clinical expertise that creates a dynamic supervisor. The goal of supervision is to assist the individual to take appropriate clinical and human action. The solving of problems is based not only on the application of rules and regulations but also on "situational thinking." One looks at the human situation that triggered reactions. For instance, one collects facts and analyzes how people behaved, what their needs were, what happened, what seemed to precipitate the incident, and what were the positive learnings from this incident that can prevent a recurrence. Decision is then made on the best method for handling the situation, which involves people as well as rules.

Who Is the Adult Learner?

We have noted that the most important goals of supervision are developmental and educative. The focus of all educational activities is centered on the needs, motivations, and psychology of the learner. Although the supervisor does have some responsibility for teaching the nursing student (a youth learner), she is concerned for the most part with the teaching of personnel, patients, and family members who are adult learners. Educators have identified differences in these two types of learners. The adult learner brings a variety of life experiences which by their very nature have helped him to know more than the youth learner. These life experiences have caused the individual to develop attitudes and perspectives which should dictate the method and content of the supervisor's plan. The adult learner has a practical, "here and now" goal; he is interested and motivated by what will help him achieve his life goals through his job. The youth learner, on the other hand, has a non-life-oriented goal; he is academically oriented toward knowledge which will be applied later when he becomes a member of the work force of society. In each twenty-four hours, the adult learner assumes many roles in society with the concomitant status, expectations, responsibilities inherent therein. These roles are associated with adulthood, and therefore the individual has a self image consistent with adulthood. Anything that shatters this image or reduces it to a childlike one sets off a chain of attitudes and behaviors which act as barriers to learning.

Maslow ranks the basic human motivational needs from low to high as follows: physical needs, safety needs, social needs, self-actualization. Those needs are motivational forces for life activities. Most hospital personnel have had the two lower needs met. It is true that the minimum level in terms of individual satisfaction varies with individuals, but basically food and housing needs are generally satisfied above the hardship level. Therefore, the higher needs—social and self-actualization—are stronger motivational forces in the adult learner. An understanding of how these needs motivate individuals to learn and change is essential for the success of the supervisor in her teaching. The field of psychology has shown the importance of building on past associations (life experiences). The adult is constantly incorporating new experiences and relating them to past ones, then reorganizing the whole. A ward aide who has cared for a sick mother has had similar activities to those on her job. The supervisor as teacher can utilize this to advantage.

The adult learner in the hospital situation is interested not in preparing for a new job but in improving his present job performance so that his needs for recognition, acceptance, and self-actualization will be met. Teaching must be so carried out that he sees the value of change from his own viewpoint. He is a practical person who is task-centered but still wants to understand the "why." Theory for the adult learner must be readily understood to have direct relationship to the realities of the job.

The Teaching Process: Formal and Informal

The teaching activities of the supervisor fall into two main types: formal and informal. Formal teaching may be defined as that which is preplanned to meet one or more specific objectives having to do with improved knowledge and performance of personnel, or to help the patient cope with his illness. Informal, or incidental, teaching is done when the need for it is demonstrated in the nursing situation. It is not preplanned and is done on the spot.

The type of teaching is determined through the teacher's assessment of the situation in terms of the learner, his specific need for teaching, and the pressures of the environment at the moment. In many cases informal teaching proves to be the most effective and appropriate; in almost all situations both formal and informal teaching are used. Sometimes the informal type is employed to supplement and enforce the formal one.

Most nurses, because of their life experience, are more knowledgeable in the techniques of formal teaching. Although they have been learners in informal teaching situations, they may not have been aware of the teaching process. For this reason supervisors are likely to assume that essential changes in performance call for correction, not teaching. The overtones of discipline and censure influence a re-education. If the supervisor sees the worker as a culprit caught while she is doing something wrong and treats her as a child, she shatters the latter's image of adulthood and sets up a chain of reactions—embarrassment, resentment, rebellion—which act as barriers to improvement. Educational psychologists have found that even in teaching children punishment does not always bring about permanent change. When its painfulness has worn off, frequently the inadequate performance reoccurs. No permanent change in behavior can be effected unless the learner understands why she should behave differently. For the same reason the adult learner needs to know why she performed in an unacceptable fashion. Communication of this knowledge must occur in a climate so free of censure that she can "hear" without mobilizing her defenses. She is then psychologically free to understand and accept the need to modify a specific behavior.

Important to incidental teaching in the work situation is the recognition of the quality of a relationship which enables the teacher to teach and the learner to learn. The human-relation skills of the teacher are of paramount importance in establishing a two-way meaningful relationship; an atmosphere of acceptance, mutual respect, and collaboration is essential.

The two-way relationship also opens communication, which is the essence of teaching. If the individual is to be moved toward change, there must be shared understanding of goals and expectations. Of course, to communicate effectively we must know the background and personalities of those whom we wish to influence. This understanding helps the teacher (supervisor) to predict reactions of the worker and to construct a learning situation tailored to her needs.

Situational Thinking

The total situation in which the worker performs influences how, when, and what is to be taught. For instance, a supervisor may observe a nurse carrying out a procedure in an atypical way. The situation may have dictated modification of the prescribed method. If the modification was wrong, teaching will focus on how it could have been made more effectively, rather than insisting that the usual procedure has no alternative.

A hectic, chaotic, busy period is not the time to pull the worker out of the situation in order to teach her. She is not psychologically ready since she is absorbed with many demands being placed on her. The wise teacher moves into the situation, gives her a hand, and directs by example. Therefore, the supervisor, as a teacher, must be a "situational thinker."

Another advantage to informal teaching is that the social distance between learner and teacher is reduced. When formal teaching is planned, a class is scheduled; the learner enters a classroom environment in which the roles of teacher and learner are clearly evident. In incidental teaching, the roles and processes are not so discernible and the distance barrier is reduced.

Successful incidental teaching demands much of the teacher. She must give constantly of herself, be conscious of the need for teaching so that she can take advantage of the opportunities, and be flexible in her method and approach. However, we cannot imagine a more stimulating way of teaching. The rewards are high in terms of mutual growth and meaningful relationship.

The Democratic Trend

The acknowledged trend from authoritarian to collaborative supervision has several variants. The supervisor may cling to the traditional "boss" concept at one end of the spectrum, or may leave decision-making to her group at the other end. Or she may adopt a compromise position somewhere along the line between the two.

Supervisory behavior has been classified by Tannenbaum and Schmidt * according to the the following continuum:

1. The supervisor identifies a problem, chooses her solution, and reports her decision to the subordinates for implementation. No opportunity is given for direct participation in the decision-making process.

2. Instead of simply announcing her decision, the supervisor tries to persuade her subordinates to adopt it. If she encounters resistance, she may indicate what the employees have to gain from the decision.

3. In addition to seeking acceptance of her ideas, the supervisor invites questions so that her subordinates can better understand what she is trying to accomplish; in this way the implications of her decision are explored more fully by her and her group.

4. The supervisor presents a tentative decision, having retained the initiative for identifying and diagnosing the problem. She says in effect: "What do you have to say about this plan? I'll appreciate your frank reactions but will make the final decision."

5. The supervisor identifies the problem but gives the subordinates the first chance to suggest their own solutions. She thus in-increases her own repertoire of possible solutions, capitalizing on the knowledge and experience of persons on the firing line. The supervisor then selects what she considers the most promising solution.

6. The supervisor passes to the group (possibly including herself as a member) the right to make decisions, but only after defining the problem and the boundaries within which the decision must be made. An example is the handling of a hospital parking problem.

7. The group identifies and diagnoses the problem, develops alter-

* Robert Tannenbaum and Warren H. Schmidt, "How to Choose a Leadership Pattern," *Harvard Business Review,* XXXVI (March–April, 1958), 95–101.

native solutions, and decides on one or more of them. The only limits imposed on the group are those laid down by its boss's superior. If the boss takes part in decision-making, he attempts to do so with no more authority than any other member. Most importantly, he commits himself in advance to implementing whatever decision the group makes.

In summary, at the boss-centered end of the continuum the emphasis is on the supervisor—her interests, attitudes, and feelings. As one moves toward the subordinate-centered end, the focus is increasingly on the subordinates—what they are interested in, how they look at things, how they feel about them.

In conclusion, it should be realized that the successful supervisor can't be primarily characterized either as a strong leader or as a permissive one. She should rather be defined as one who can accurately assess the forces that determine her behavior at any given time and can behave accordingly.

4

WHAT IS THE CASE METHOD?

Principles and Practices

Epictetus on Philosophy:
> Here is the beginning of philosophy:
> a recognition of the conflicts between men,
> a search for their cause,
> a condemnation of mere opinion . . .
> and the *discovery of a standard of judgment*.
> *Discourses*, First Century A.D.

At this point, the reader may say that it's fine to theorize about dynamic, participative supervision, but "it doesn't apply to my experience." She then reviews her own supervisory practices in the hospital and despairingly concludes that "you can't teach an old dog . . . , you can't make a silk purse. . . ."

Our experience with a large number of in-service training programs has continually reinforced our belief that behavior can be changed. The supervisors who attended our sessions over a long period of time recognized the need to change their supervisory behavior. They eagerly searched for new methods that would equip them to help others to change, while being aware that they as change agents must be willing to change too. We are convinced that any method used to educate toward change must be collaborative and participative. Then, this method is not only a teaching-learning tool, but in fact it becomes a way of behaving. The case method is a most effective mode of promoting learning and change. The case method in in-service training may be defined as a device for educating supervisory personnel through group learning for the integration of individual needs and organizational aims. The goal is improvement in performance through individual growth. This method is most successful when the leader fashions her approach and methods out of an understanding of the adult learner. Indeed, in-service training *is* adult education. To grasp this truth let us review some of the differences between the learning psychology of the youth and that of the adult.

Youth and Adult Learners

There are striking contrasts between youth and adult learners. In the first place, youth does not have a here-and-now motivation; the practical application of learnings is postponed, and they are regarded as preparation for the future. Adults, on the other hand, want to use their learnings to solve particular life problems which confront them. They tend to have clearer and more immediate purposes for learning.

Youths are in a dependent, receiving role, whereas adults must be dynamically involved in the learning process. The case method is admirably suited to meet the needs of the mature individual, since it involves him actively with his peers and the group leader in a joint process of investigation and analysis. The authority-obedience and examination-evaluation syndromes of undergraduate education are eliminated in the effort to encourage collaborative thinking in a permissive climate. The goal of adult education is to develop the capacity for self-initiated learning. Programs for adults are now based on individual and social problems instead of traditional academic principles of subject organization.

Adult learners want to talk things over, to see all the angles, to clarify their thinking, and to reason about things, rather than to acquire knowledge for its own sake. They seek to mobilize all previous knowledge and experience to apply to the immediate problem.

Briefly, the case method creates a practice laboratory where the participants expose their ideas and test them in the cross fire of analysis and diagnosis. They are provided with the raw material of a concrete case which they analyze collaboratively to find responsible ways of resolving the problem. The aim is to evolve a process of thinking rather than to impart information, to illuminate the complex forces underlying a problem situation.

The case method is one approach to overcome the limitations of traditional in-service education. It conforms to sound psychological principles and learning theories. This method gives the individual the ego satisfactions of being involved; of being recognized for all contributions, not just the "good" ones; of being free to disagree with no risk of rejection; and of having the opportunity to reveal and reconcile differences instead of repressing them.

The Cause-Result Approach

An acknowledged principle of human behavior underlies the case method, namely that there are many causes behind every action. What is aimed at is the development of a multi-cause-result approach to problem analysis instead of the common blame-responsibility syndrome. The discussants are stimulated by the leader to examine the variables that influence a seemingly simple situation. This shakes up a two-value orientation and prevents a doctrinaire approach to problem-solving. Yes, there may be two sides to every problem, but how complex the sides are! Erecting a dichotomy oversimplifies. "No halfway about truth" may be a valid philosophical position, but it is not effective in problem-solving when interpretation of facts ("truth") is critical. The case method is not intended to illustrate definitive "good" or "bad" practices but to represent reality. Participants are encouraged to interpret concrete situations, to make inferences and judgments, and to suggest possible actions. Active, dynamic involvement replaces a routinized, passive approach. The emphasis is on joint analysis of the many factors, supported conclusions, and formulation of imaginative, realistic solutions that can be translated into action. The group members learn to go from specific instances to general conclusions.

The case method also facilitates and increases communication, which is the essence of teaching. The psychological distance between learner and leader is less than when formal instruction is carried out. This democratic climate encourages new relationships between leader and member, as well as between member and member. All contributions are equally valuable, and this exchange provides a learning-from-each-other opportunity.

Another important learning principle which the case method recognizes is that wisdom can't be told, sold, or taught. No lecture on improving sensitivity, understanding, insight, or judgment will suffice by itself. People must "grow their own." Educational psychologists point out that effective learning involves an active, dynamic process in the learner. This enables the individual to modify and alter the way in which he perceives a situation. Such learning is more meaningful and permanent than that gained from "being told."

Participants Are Sensitized

One of the most significant functions of the case method is sensitization of participants to their own attitudes and behavior, so that they can perceive how these hinder or contribute to problem-solving. In studying actual on-the-job problems in a permissive atmosphere of free inquiry, the discussants begin to recognize the limits of their private perception and the need for breaking through their emotional barriers—fears, prejudices, blind spots—which block objectivity of judgment and have a harmful effect on human relationships. They also develop an awareness that dearly held assumptions and values may cause one to view a situation through a distorting lens. The defense of one's own view may prevent accepting the values of others. A better understanding of our own limitations and biases may make us less condemnatory of others' ideas and more empathic with their attitudes and objectives.

We agree with the observation that differences of opinion and ideas are most likely to stimulate innovative solutions to problem-solving, and that polite "reasonableness" tends to suppress creativity. If the leader encourages a respect for disagreement during the discussion, soon the climate will be safe for members to express unpopular and unique opinions and attitudes. Disagreements must not be seen as an attack, but often the beginning of innovation. Dissonance is not disloyalty but often is a break-through to reduce a trend to conformity. When the leader accepts (not necessarily *agrees* with) each contribution and shows respect for the importance of the individual's feeling and comments, the climate of discussion becomes safe for diversity. In fact, the leader can actively encourage and stimulate differences of opinions by asking these kinds of questions:

Does someone think of a different method or plan?
Who can expand that idea?
Let's try to think of the direct opposite of that suggestion.
What would be the ideal way of handling the situation?
What concerns or frustrates you the most about this problem?
Let's list the advantages and disadvantages of the solutions discussed so far.

During case discussion there is full freedom to criticize and challenge the opinions of others. Skills are developed in reconciling opposing viewpoints. This leads to an increased capacity for open, authentic collaborative relationships, even to a new style of working with and through others. The mutual recrimination that has often beset problem-solving in the past is replaced by mutual understanding.

Heretofore, problem-solving has frequently been an undisciplined process involving quick, impressionistic rule-of-thumb solutions. Now the goal is to increase the depth of ways of examining situations, to see the distortions of surface perceptions—the denials, evasions, and misleading single-cause-and-effect reasoning which make so-called "solutions" fail.

What Is a Case?

The case is an accurate description of what happened in a real life situation, in terms of people, place, and time. The leader and participants must realize that neither in the case nor on the job are all the facts available. The challenge is to arrive at feasible solutions in spite of the insufficiency of available facts.

In the beginning it is better if the cases come from situations outside the institution. The participants will be able to analyze the case and learn from it without the barriers of personal biases or loyalties. As they learn to focus on the diagnosis of the case instead of assessing blame, it is hoped that the skills of collaborative analysis, developed by using the cases presented in this book, can be transferred to the analysis of their own on-the-job problems.

Participative Learning Through Group Discussion

One-man solutions, like one-man discoveries, are no longer appropriate in a complex hospital organization. In the case method of in-service training the learning needed for reaching wise solutions becomes a democratic three-way social transaction: leader-to-learner, learner-to-leader, and learner-to-learner.

By examining the relationship forces operating in the group, its members become aware of interpersonal and group dynamics which can help or hinder collaborative effort. They are no longer passive observers but active participants in the learning process. Increasingly, too, they develop new ways of accepting and responding to each other, and realize that the discussion of any on-the-job situation must include consideration of others' emotional as well as rational actions, that people are psychological and logical. The interpersonal dynamics of attitudes, sentiments, and prejudices are often more significant than the actual event.

What is required, then, is the pooling of individual resources, experiences, judgments, assumptions, and attitudes, without emphasis on the need for agreement. This is followed by the collaborative analysis of key elements of problems, with fundamental questions raised, a critical spirit of inquiry encouraged, and useful principles developed. A continuous process of free inquiry is fostered, with deviant and divergent ideas expressed, examined, reality-tested, and if necessary modified.

It should be realized that even the "best" single member of a group sees a given situation through the prism of her own personality and experience. In group discussion the participants see how differently each perceives the same set of conditions. The individual who contributes a solution becomes conscious that others' ideas may be as good as or better than her own, and that often sounder decisions can be made through joint effort. Discourse and disputation help to discover nuances in a situation. They lead to the habit of consulting, sharing in the decision-making process, and reconciling divergent ideas. Free discussion helps in correcting distortions and makes for greater objectivity. By contributing a variety of "know-how," the discussants gain a new vantage point for liberating, enriching, or modifying useful conjectures. The case system helps members develop an awareness that many alternatives exist for the interpretation and resolution of a problem. They learn that effectiveness in solving a dilemma requires examination of several alternatives—they can't "know 'em all."

A graphic way to illustrate how knowledge is increased through the exchange of ideas is to compare the process with a money exchange. If A and B swap a dollar, each has only one; if they exchange ideas, each now has two—the original thought and a new one.

5

WHAT, WHY, AND HOW OF THE SEMINAR

Administrative Clearance for the Program

Any in-service program is an integrated, continuing program which requires the cooperation of many people in different departments; for this reason it must have the understanding, approval, and support of administration, both for the program itself and for the possible transfer of learnings from the seminar to the job. The training given will be successful if the organization supports the new patterns of supervison that result.

The proper planning of a case-method seminar is essential for its effectiveness. The active support of administration is indispensable for the success of any in-service program, and concurrence in regard to goals is the surest guaranty of this support. For this reason it is well for the leader to discuss in detail her objectives and over-all plans with the director of nurses and her assistants before the seminar opens.

Enrollment is voluntary, and personnel at all supervisory levels are eligible—not only the actual supervisors but everyone who assists in carrying out the supervisory process. The membership should be under fifteen, since larger numbers inhibit free and frequent interaction.

Widely separated meetings are less effective than frequent ones. The model schedule calls for two-hour weekly meetings continued for at least 15 weeks—a minimum total of 30 hours.

Who Should Lead?

Feelings and opinions are recruited, the heart is enlarged and the human mind is developed only by the reciprocal influence of men upon one another.

Alexis de Tocqueville, *Democracy in America*

The leader of this case-method seminar may be either an outside trainer or a member of the hospital line or staff personnel. There are compelling reasons for preferring the latter.

In the first place, the concepts and process of participative supervision and those of leadership in the seminar complement each other; both processes are based on the same philosophy. Second, when a supervisor leads the discussion, both she and the participants are likely to learn more about their own values and interpersonal relationships.

In keeping with the principles of adult education the leader and the group members are co-learners. This relationship of collaboration reduces the likelihood of learning and teaching one kind of behavior and skills in the meetings, another kind on the job. Having a member of the inside personnel act as leader makes it possible to reduce the extreme frustration and confusion that arise when new learnings gained from an in-service training experience are not in harmony with existing policy and philosophy. New insights must be usable beyond the situation in which the learning occurred. An *inside* leader can reinforce the transfer and application of new behavior and attitudes.

Finally, the supervisor acting as leader is in a position to encourage discussion of on-the-job problems which have hitherto been ignored because she and they were "too busy" to work collaboratively or had little freedom or desire to do so.

How to Lead

The leader must remind herself that she is approaching a group of adult learners whose motivational needs are primarily pragmatic and self-actualizing. She should understand how these needs influence learning and willingness to change.

If the leader accepts and applies the supervisory concepts of shared goals and joint problem-solving, the forces of participation will be released. As the members come to accept responsibility to contribute to the discussion, their motivation to learn will replace compliance, conformity, and reliance on tried-and-true methods. An important characteristic of the case system is that the leader must inspire activity and partnership in the joint process of learning. Both leader and members have the same case to analyze; thus it follows that there is equal opportunity to contribute. Remember that a good teacher challenges the learner and that to challenge is not to win a point, not to control, but rather to encourage the participant on his own terms.

In opening the seminar, the leader may make some of the following introductory comments:

Developing skills in human relations is not a neat process of acquiring techniques; rather it is a way of learning to increase our sensitivity and awareness of a concrete situation and then trying to improve our response to it. These skills are not effectively talked about; they are something to be practiced.

or

In these meetings, instead of my exhorting about your attitudes, reactions, and values or theorizing about motivations, personalities, and supervisory practices, we shall analyze specific situations in a spirit of give and take.

or

I shall try to help you look at these cases from the viewpoint of the persons involved in them, to examine the causes of their behavior instead of blaming them.

or

As the meetings proceed we will, I hope, not only recognize facts but will also use our imagination to penetrate beneath them in our search for answers to problems. In this way creative sparks will be struck off which will in turn generate new concepts and fresh approaches.

After everyone has had time to read the case, the leader can start the discussion by asking such questions as these:

What do you think is the problem here?
Who has a different opinion?
What is going on in this situation?
Who is willing to start the discussion by telling us what the heart of the problem is as you see it?

As the exchange of opinions and ideas gets under way, the leader may ask (not necessarily in sequence):

What do you think are the issues involved here?
What are some of the pressures you feel are creating this problem?
What principles are involved?
What additional information would you like to obtain before taking any action?
What would you do in this situation if you were in charge?
How would you go about solving the problem?
Does someone want to comment on that?
How can we apply this idea?
What are some resources that might remedy the situation?

Use summarizing questions; for example, "Do I understand that you feel . . . ," "Then I gather you favor . . . ."
Avoid asking questions that are easily answered by "yes" or "no."
Questioning is really a diagnostic method that can help to clarify and define issues, facts, feelings, and relationships. Remember than an effective questioner is also a good listener.
You may want to try another way of conducting the discussion. After the group has read the case (aloud or privately), ask for

general impressions, which you put on the board. Divide the group into several small units to continue the discussion for 20 to 30 minutes. Ask a spokesman from each subgroup to report the members' suggested solutions and alternatives. After writing these on the blackboard, alongside the first impressions, continue discussion and analysis with the total group. You will likely see many shifts in points of view from the first impressions recorded on the board.

Setting the Climate

The first meeting may present special problems. One that the leader might encounter is the attitude of the participants toward her. If this is their first experience with the case method, some of them may carry into the opening meeting feelings, relationships, or unresolved conflicts that have developed on the job. Associated with these may be anxiety as to the leader's competence and motivation.

A frequent source of tension and constraint is the result of previous conditioning of group members to rigid supervision from above, with limited opportunity for individual responsibility and initiative. For this reason they may be reluctant to accept the leader's invitation to full participation.

Furthermore, most learners have become used to expecting answers and solutions from higher authorities. As a result they may be suspicious of proposals to do their own problem-solving and may show little appreciation and even distrust of team effort. If, however, the climate is permissive and the leader's attitude is one of acceptance, and if she succeeds in demonstrating that she and the participants are co-learners, they will join the collaboration and soon be excited by the sparks thrown off when mind rubs against mind.

In order to lessen dependence on and deference to authority, the leader should aim at developing in the discussants a new sense of personal reponsibility and commitment. This is one way of replacing ingrained compliance with independent thought and action.

Another difficulty may arise from the fact that the case method of learning is quite different from participants' previous experience.

They may be accustomed to the usual procedure of memorizing and storing knowledge in specific content areas. Also, since the case method stresses the process of learning through peer collaboration, members may feel frustrated when asked to deal with nebulous situations out of which they must make sense. Furthermore, discussions reveal so many contrasting points of view that frustration may develop because there is no simple answer to the situation under discussion.

It takes a while for new participants to "catch" the spirit of the case system with its inquiry, weighing of pro's and con's, assessing facts and feelings, exploring causal relationships, its emphasis on active, unguarded participation. Therefore, one case a week should not be rigidly scheduled. Often groups need to spend more than one session analyzing a case.

Sometimes there is an expectation of acquiring facts and packaged solutions to supervisory problems. An important learning the case method provides is that often there is no one final, unequivocal solution to a human dilemma. On the other hand, some situations are capable of several acceptable alternatives—others are not capable of even one satisfactory resolution. But in all these events, the emphasis is on developing skills in the process of thinking analytically (in a joint relationship) in a new situation with a new combination of issues.

More About the Leader

The case discussion leader is a liberator, not a commander. Her primary responsibility is to encourage participative learning and mutual problem-solving in a confidential, nonjudgmental climate. An atmosphere of this kind encourages creative expresssion instead of submissiveness, dependence, and repression. It fosters freedom of opinion and dissent, and the feeling that one has a right to be wrong. Members say what they feel, not what they think they ought to say. They are at liberty to express ideas and attitudes without fear of hostile criticism and isolation, but they are discouraged from relying on "tried-and-true" methods of problem-solving.

The leader strictly avoids didactic teaching; her aim is to elicit opinions, not to transmit accepted theories and techniques. Nor will she use her status or authority to coerce or negate opinions. Instead, she supports the group as it learns to define, assess, and diagnose human relations problems objectively and rationally, distinguishing fact from opinion. The group members are encouraged to practice making assumptions and hypotheses and reality-testing them; to challenge one another's views and examine their own opinions, reversing and revising them if necessary.

The leader also summarizes discussions and clarifies issues. If she asks questions, it is to define the issue, not to examine the person. She directs discussions away from impressionistic judgments and toward complete analysis of problems, keeping the focus of attention on cases instead of on personalities.

In establishing and maintaining a permissive climate the leader should be neutral but not detached. Neither censor nor critic, she avoids placing the group members on the defensive. Respecting all statements even though they seem to her incorrect or irrelevant, she fosters fresh exploration, remembering that disapproval kills discussion, disagreement stimulates it. The leader may state her own views but should invite the same critical appraisal of them that the participants give to each others' ideas.

In participative learning the group members realize that many of the questions raised are not simple and susceptible to pat answers but are many-sided and complex. For some people problem-solving consists in working obsessively with habitual or "first" ideas, however fruitless they may be; such ideas tend to be self-perpetuating. Others are prone to erect dichotomies—the either-or, win-or-lose, right-or-wrong orientation. A change in these modes of thinking occurs when discussants understand the need of proposing and testing alternatives in order to prevent an impasse.

Case discussion also trains people to use conflict situations creatively. Conflict is inherent in any dynamic organization and is an inescapable corollary of institutional change. What is is needed is not to repress conflict but to devise ways of resolving it. Both complementary and conflicting views are fundamental elements for the solution of human relations problems.

Specifically, the behavior of the leader is as follows:

1. She assumes responsibility for seeing that the discussion is pertinent to the case. However, she allows the group to give direction to the discussion as long as it is relevant, though she had not foreseen this approach in her case planning.
2. She observes interaction between group members, draws out the retiring and prevents domination by others.
3. She asks questions to assist the group to advance toward conclusions, and then to test feasibility and implications of decisions.
4. She avoids taking the role of the expert by referring questions directed to her back to the group.
5. She clarifies and gives information that group members may not have.
6. She may list significant facts, issues, recommendations on the board for continual study and reference of the group.
7. She avoids approval or disapproval of contributions, condescension, sarcasm, personal cross-examination, self-approval.
8. She may voice her own opinions and share her knowledge, but avoids domination.
9. She prevents blame assessment on characters in the case by focusing on the processes and action in the *case*.
10. If the group is not moving forward in the discussion, she may by astute questions have the members look at why they are "frozen."
11. She stimulates and guides opinions, instead of waiting for fuzzy attitudes to congeal.

Do's and Don'ts

In conclusion we suggest some do's and don'ts for effective leadership in the case method:

DO'S

1. Help the members to ask better questions; for example, "Why did that occur?" instead of "Who was at fault?"
2. Aid the members to recognize their own attitudes, biases, and

feelings. Urge them to examine their own behavior by looking at the values and emotions underlying their suggestions, just as they try to understand the "why" of behavior of the subjects in the case. In this way the emotional and interpersonal elements of the "here and now" are explored along with the "there and then" of the case.

3. Help the group to probe beyond the "charm school" approach of pat answers and moralistic platitudes, such as "Apply the Golden Rule" or "You can catch more flies . . . ."

4. Help the discussants to determine "what is going on in this situation."

5. Bear in mind that your functions are to raise questions that others neglect, to provoke differing opinions, to prevent acceptance of unsupported views, to encourage challenges, to integrate ideas, to accept interpretations with which you may disagree.

6. If someone is making a long statement, interrupt by asking for some explicit point.

7. Pin down the maker of generalizations, such as "most people," "all supervisors," "everybody does."

8. Guard against "good" or "bad," "fish or cut bait" solutions.

9. If there is a debate about the meaning of words, probe for the feelings behind them.

10. If a discussant is inclined to reject evidence because it does not fit into her preconceived notion, point out that it may still have value in solving the problem.

11. Help members to avoid the pitfall of waving aside complexity in their hope for a few clear-cut rules. Complexity is inescapably inherent in most human relations problems. Point out that attempts to oversimplify a situation will prevent reaching an understanding of it.

12. Guard against the group's accepting solutions that place blame on a single individual and that suggest he be fired or transferred.

13. Watch for snap judgments, global solutions, and "instant" psychiatric labels like "Oh, he's psychotic."

14. Ask about the "how" as well as the "what" of actions. This will evoke a variety of responses and assumptions about appropriate behavior in the situation.
15. Summarize discussion periodically.

DON'TS

1. Don't insist on having the last word.
2. Don't talk more than the participants do. "The less the teacher 'teaches', the more the learner learns."
3. Don't pronounce how anyone *should* feel, but respond to the authentic feelings she is expressing.
4. Don't allow an inference or conjecture to pass as a fact.
5. Don't give in to an urge to advise anyone how to feel, act, or behave.
6. Don't think you know the "best" solution. Keep the open mind you encourage others to cultivate. Fresh points of view have a two-way direction.
7. Remember that you do not control the "right" answers.
8. Your approval of a contribution should not be a reward nor your disapproval a punishment.

Goals of Analysis

The analytic process is directed both at the individual's own judgments and at the problem to be solved. Personal judgments are likely to be impressionistic and based on the immediate emotional response. Unless one's "answer" is analyzed, it tends to be self-validating—that is, to make the judgment consistent with the situation—whereas the need is to transcend the limits of immediate perception. Self-analysis goes beyond the instantaneous reaction.

It should be realized that often long-term benefits from analyzing a problem are more important than solving it. Whereas the solution for one problem will probably never fit another, the process, the method employed, can be applied to each new situation. The case method teaches the process of thinking in new and unfamiliar situations—to be resourceful and courageous in new approaches. Knowledge and logic must supplement intuition.

Group analysis is needed to ferret out the problem; it must also examine relationships, policies, and personalities before responsible action is decided upon. Analysis of facts, inferences, and feelings is the basis for suggesting courses of action. There is also a need to reality-test possible solutions by asking such questions as "What is to be done?" "By whom?" "What reactions will this course of action produce in the system?" If the analysis is superficial or unrealistic, such reality-testing by the group will reveal its inadequacy.

The chief benefit of joint analysis is the release of creative thinking by moving away from right-wrong, win-lose, black-white orientation, which is dysfunctional; it breaks the rigid, stereotyped patterns of problem-solving.

Here are some actual responses which show failure to perceive the complexity of human relation situations:

Stereotyped thinking about people and situations:

The loud-mouthed type
The kind of person who . . .
All hospital employees . . .

The two-value approach (either-or analysis):

There are only two possibilities.
There are three ways of approaching this.
It's either right or wrong, logical or illogical.

Oversimplified cause-and-effect analysis:

This is *just* a communication problem.
Insecurity is the cause.
Not enough efficiency.
Everyone knows that . . .

Blame-pinning

He's the cause of it all.
It's one man's responsibility.
The problem would never have arisen if he hadn't . . .

Labeling

An inferiority complex.
A joker, a playboy.
An obvious thing.

Evaluation

In-service training by the case method is fundamentally a process of changing people's knowledge, skills, attitudes, and behavior in the direction desired by the individuals and the organization to further the objectives of nursing care. A critical factor in the success of this kind of program is the potential transferability of the experience—the direct relationship of the seminar to hospital life. The insights, skills, and learnings must not remain outside the mainstream of the hospital.

Evaluation of such training, broadly speaking, attempts to answer the following questions:

1. To what extent have the desired changes been brought about?
2. How well have the trainees learned what was being taught?
3. Have they applied these learnings?
4. How can the training process be improved?

When and how to make these assessments are difficult questions. There is no dogmatic prescription in regard to timing or method, for needs, both organizational and personal, undergo constant alteration and are influenced by many factors. This has been demonstrated by reaction questionnaires and discussions (both formal and informal) with participants following the conclusion of previous seminars. Because of these perpetual changes and variety of influences it is necessary to keep revising specific training activities and goals, and to see that they are always related to actual problems.

Another difficulty of evaluation lies in determining the goals of growth for members of case-method seminars. Not all individuals are equally able to change; each has different problems, different strengths and weaknesses. For some persons learning is immediate; others require varying periods of incubation. Also criteria as to how much insight a member can stand are lacking; little is known about evaluating insights or about the processes by which they are internalized.

One of the hoped-for outcomes is that the group members will identify areas in which they want more information. This need can serve to motivate group exploration and discussion of literature. This will lead to richer analysis of the cases. For example, the preliminary discussions will expose such areas as bringing about change, communications barriers, improving organizational effectiveness, and evaluating personnel performance and nursing care. A little detective work in the book review sections of the nursing journals, the promotional materials from publishers, and our references will reveal good sources for discussion. It is surprising how much basic material dealing with these areas is available in the public libraries. It may not be identified under nursing, but the principles and theories are applicable even though many people think "nursing is different."

Ongoing evaluation of each session by the leader and group members can be done by posing the following questions:

What was the climate of the group?
  Did members defer to the leader?
  Was there freedom to express disagreement?
  Did members avoid differences?
  Did members allow minority opinions?

How well were members listening to each other?
  Were comments relevant to preceding remarks?
  Was there willingness to consider other ideas?
  Was there evidence of members blindly defending their own position (open versus closed mind)?
  Did anyone suggest alternative solutions?

What other means could have been used to help the group to reach agreements and decisions?

Postseminar evaluation forms (anonymous) will yield data on the feelings of participants, the development of interpersonal and interdepartmental relationships, transferability of learnings, and suggestions for program improvement. These data, however, can be considered only suggestive, not conclusive.

From Seminar to Job

Perhaps the most vital function of the case method is to provide a framework for dealing with supervisory problems on the job. In the seminar the participants discover significant principles and processes to be applied to these problems, in addition to devising solutions for specific situations.

The carry-over of behavioral changes induced in the seminar begins even before the meetings are concluded. Give-and-take in discussions helps people to deal cooperatively with each other in the work situations. If group training produces individual satisfactions and insights, the members will be more competent to handle stubborn and harassing supervisory problems.

A significant aspect of the case-method seminar is that it creates an axis for new relationships between members. Through a free exchange of views individuals turn new facets of themselves to each other. Because this kind of interaction is free of typical organizational restraints, the transfer of new working relationships can have important organizational consequences. The seminar members reinvest themselves in their jobs and interpersonal relationships. Supervisors now examine objectively the patterns of their resistance to change built into their own organizational methods. Rigid practices that have become institutionalized without any basic policy rationale are studied or even changed. The supervisor finds that she can be more effective in dealing with others and their problems. The blame syndrome is diminished, for the participants realize by personal experience that understanding another's behavior can eliminate the necessity for censure. They learn to place self-and-other problems in a larger perspective, thus reducing breakdowns in communication which cause relationship failures.

It should be noted that the case method does not magically *change* hospital experiences and problems; it helps to alter the ways in which individuals interpret and resolve them. Old "facts" take on new meanings, so that subsequent problems are perceived with improved insights.

Furthermore, the new relationship of cooperation in analyzing and solving problems may reduce disturbed relationships between departments as well as between staff members; the result is better understanding of factional, interdepartmental, and intradepartmental problems. The pooling of opinions, facts, and ideas, the collaborative problem-solving attitudes, may become habit-forming and be transferred from the seminar to the hospital.

A Sample Analysis

Here is a demonstration case which can be used with the group —possibly at the start.

A Terminal Interview with Mrs. May, R.N.*

Returning from lunch one day, Mrs. Doris Wechsler, the personnel director at Blake General Hospital in Philadelphia, met Miss Cecilia Joyce, the head of the Nursing Service, in the elevator.

"Say, I understand Mrs. May, down in out-patient, has decided to quit," Mrs. Wechsler remarked.

"Yes," replied Miss Joyce. "She handed in her resignation yesterday, effective in two weeks. I don't know whether to be glad or sorry!"

"My secretary says she was in this morning trying to make an appointment with me," Mrs. Wechsler observed. "You know, she's often come in to discuss her ideas with me. I thought I'd see her if it's all right with you."

"Sure! I wish you could find out something!" exclaimed Miss Joyce. "This case defeats me entirely. She's a good nurse, one of our own graduates. Yet, somehow, she never seemed to get onto the way things go around here. I feel I failed too, somehow, in helping her."

"O.K." said Mrs. Wechsler. "I'll see her. If we can get an idea of

* Permission was granted by the Board of Trustees of Boston University to modify and reprint this case contained in *Case Studies in Nursing Service Administration*, Volume I, compiled by the faculty and graduate students of Boston University School of Nursing, and copyrighted 1954 by the Board of Trustees of Boston University. Copies of the unmodified case may be obtained through the Boston University Book Store (14/MGTIMM4). The assignment to group discussants is that of the authors.

what she thinks her troubles are we may at least help her to avoid the same sort of difficulties in the next place she works."

Mrs. Wechsler made an appointment with Mrs. May for the following day at 5 P.M., which was "after hours" for both of them. When Mrs. May appeared, the personnel director invited her to sit down, thinking as she did so, that Mrs. May always looked and acted much younger than her 31 years.

"Well, I suppose you know I've finally quit," began Mrs. May without preliminary. "I could talk all night about the reasons, but when I begin to bore you, just shut me off! I've just got to unload to somebody!"

She then said she didn't know where to begin, there was so much to tell. But perhaps the best place to start was with how the nurses felt about the administration, the nursing office. She said, "The people in that office are all old maids. If they ever had any love-life, it was well suppressed years ago, and they don't want anyone else to have any. Their supervision goes into every area of a nurse's life.

"It is the little things that count, and it continues all the time you are associated with the hospital, not only as a student. When we were students, we more or less expected to be disciplined. I graduated in 1939—a long time ago—and things have changed a lot since then. It is much easier to be a student now. The cadet nurses are largely responsible for that. They wouldn't take a lot of the things that the regular students had to take in the old days. They really did a lot for the student nurses. There are more 'lates' than we ever dreamed of, and, of course, they could marry the last four months of their training, and they did usually. The students, then, don't have too tough a time, but the grads do. The nursing office never acts as if you knew anything. You are never told you did a good job. The doctors will tell you often, but never anyone in the nursing office. They will come down and find something to criticize. In fact, one supervisor whom I know was called down by the nursing office because she didn't have anything to report. She was told she was a poor supervisor if she could not find something wrong, and to go back and find it!"

Mrs. May paused only for breath. There was no need for Mrs. Wechsler to say anything to keep the interview going.

"Take the matter of coffee in the morning. Now, when you come on duty at 7, you need your coffee by 10. Everyone does it, but you have to sneak it. That isn't right. I just told one of them, 'I do it, and I'm going to continue to do it, because I feel I need it.' " Mrs. May went on for a few moments about milk and crackers being available for the nurses, but she felt she needed a pick-up—coffee rather than milk. "Boy," she exclaimed, "they really hate me around here! Oh, some of the supervisors don't, but most of them do. I get so excited about this problem, but it is really awful. Nursing isn't a profession any more!"

At this point, there was a slight pause. Mrs. Wechsler said, "I hear so much about Miss Callahan, the nursing director who retired about four years ago. Did much of this go on in her regime, too?"

Mrs. May said, "It went on, but she didn't know it. She wouldn't have liked it if she had, and when an instance did come to her attention she did something about it. Miss Callahan was different. She was very *fair*, and she was on the side of love and romance every single time. Why, we had one girl in training with us who used to come in habitually at 12:30 when we were supposed to be in at 12. She'd just go into Miss Callahan's office and bat her long lashes and say she just didn't realize that the time was going . . . and she'd get away with it; but with Miss Joyce, even when a cadet nurse went in to tell her she was getting married, she'd put her through the third degree: Is this right? Do you really think you ought to? And another thing . . . when Miss Callahan was mad, she yelled at you if she wanted to— and then it was all over. Miss Joyce and Miss Biedel don't ever raise their voices. They just hold it in for you. Neither of them is half the woman Miss Callahan was!

"But there was another thing I wanted to tell you about. They really got worried here last spring. The Head Nurse down in surgical out-patient, Suzie Shaw, was very good, one of the best we ever had. She was very well liked by the doctors and did a swell job. They have a terribly big number of patients to manage every day. I think it averages 140, and many days it goes over 200. And there is lots of quite important work done there, where the patient needs expert attention. Miss Shaw felt she couldn't carry on with her student help, and she went to the supervisor, Miss Lambert, and asked her for the part time of one graduate nurse to help her. We even knew there was a girl who wanted the job! Miss Lambert said, 'What! An out-patient department? It is the easiest thing in the world to run.' She said this without even coming down to see what the girl's problems were—that's another thing; if they'd get around this hospital and see what is going on. . . . That's why I think it is a good thing for an outsider like you to come in once in a while—somebody who isn't one of the old gang.

"Another thing Suzie objected to—there was one clerk who kept the records, and on her day off Suzie, a trained nurse, had to go in and take over the records—something any steno could do—and another nurse had to take her place. Everyone thought it was the screwiest arrangement. . . . Well, anyway, they reckoned without Miss Shaw! She handed in her resignation. Well, when Dr. Gibney (the head of out-patient) heard about it, he hit the ceiling. He went in to Miss Lambert and he told her where to head in. He told her that Miss Shaw was the 'best damn nurse' he'd ever had, and if she had asked for something, she was to get it! Well, Miss Lambert changed her attitude completely. She offered Suzie an assistant, a clerk for the day when the regular clerk was off, and even more pay, but Suzie said 'no'. One of the doctors had offered her a job in his office. More pay, better hours, and pleasant work with someone who appreciates what you're trying to do. She told Miss Lambert she hadn't asked for any of the things she wanted for herself but for the good of the patients. The nursing office still hasn't heard the end of that episode.

"There are a lot of things that they could do to make it easier, though you have said yourself you really get to love the place, and it would be so easy to remedy a lot of these things. For an example, the hours. We're supposed to get in here at 7:30. Now the patients don't start coming to out-patient until 9. So what do we do for the most part . . . read the paper, and gab. I don't get here. Everyone knows I just can't get to work on time. I got up every morning in school for three years at 6 and was everywhere on time, and I haven't done it since. It isn't as if I were relieving a night nurse. There just isn't anything to do but sit around and wait. Now is there any sense to that? They say you can read cases or correct student cases, but I can't do that the first thing in the morning. Nurses are supposed to make out their reports on lots of things the first hour, but very few do; they don't feel like it. But when I pointed out that it was ridiculous, the reply I got was, 'Mrs. May, Miss Jason and Miss Perkins who preceded you were two of the best nurses we ever had, and they thought it important to be here at 7. Do you see why you shouldn't be?'

"That's the only thing they can put down against me: that I'm late. You know they make out a kind of efficiency report on each nurse who is leaving. Mrs. Gerber, who is our direct boss, showed me the blank. It has a thousand things on it. I went over it point by point with her and said, 'This is good', 'That's unnecessary', and 'That's stupid', about different items. I told her when I got to the item about lateness, 'Well, that's the only one they can get me on here'. She said—she laughed—everyone knows I'm always late—'How about this?' pointing to a supply item. 'You let your glove count get pretty low'. Now that was what she pointed out—I let my glove count get low, once in three years! Actually, that was a time when I was on vacation, and the girl who took my place asked her what to do about gloves and she said, 'Let it go, if she could, till I came back'. So, of course, when I came back it was low. . . . But she insisted it was another time. She said I didn't order them right. Well, they get the new supply once a month and I usually order 10 pair right away (20 is the maximum you can order in the month). Most people, Mrs. Gerber said, order two or three pairs at a time all month long. Well, I think that's silly. Order them and have them. Never mind wasting time making out forms so often. It just seems stupid to me. I know Mrs. Gerber doesn't intend to make out my form until I'm gone. She hasn't said so, but I just know it.

"It's so hard to get anything here. One time a man came in from the Adirondacks who had made some very light splints for hand injuries. I thought they were grand and wanted some for my patients, so I went looking for the doctor who was head of the clinic but he wasn't around and I couldn't find an assistant, so I went to Dr. Geroux's office (the director of the hospital) and asked his secretary if she thought he'd mind talking to the man. The man was going back that night; he couldn't wait around all day for us to make up our minds. So Dr. Geroux heard us and called, 'Come in', and he and the man had a fine chat; he knew just where the place was the man came from and they had a fine time together. I got my splints, too. It was that easy. I showed them to the others the next day, and about the middle of the day the supervisor came over and said the next time I wanted supplies to come to her, not to be jumping channels. I had never even thought of *her*. By the time she'd processed something, six other places would have had the splints.

"Really, if you are so small-minded that you get upset if anyone goes around you at all, no matter what the circumstances, you must be a miserable person. . . .

"Well, have I given you some ideas? Now you can see why they have 70 beds closed in Claverley (surgical ward). There'll be more if they don't watch out. Everyone knows that Miss Biedel doesn't intend to open anything until she gets enough nurses for her pet, Brownell (private surgical wing). That's the word, if you ask for a change, you'll get Brownell—and still they build new buildings. What are they going to put in them for nurses? Even cancer is waiting now. We used to take cancer in the day it was diagnosed. Now, it has to wait several days. That may not seem like much, but it goes on with everything. We have vein cases ahead for 15 months and even two years. We have hernia and tumor operations ahead for two to three months. All these sick people who can't get in. With Blue Cross and Blue Shield they will be demanding to get in. And the old fogies better watch their step!

"Why, this place ought to be a leader. But Chicago hospitals, New York, and lots of other places are doing much better by their nurses, as to pay and everything else. I wish you'd get interested in this. I wish the public would. I wish someone would write a letter to the *Inquirer*. This is a very serious situation. And it's not only *this* hospital, though this is one of the worst.

"Say, I could talk all night, but I've got to get home and clean house. I told the minister the other day when he said he would come to call, 'Don't come till after the holidays; I have to clean up. It's a mess'. I feel much better just getting a chance to say my piece. You're the only one who ever listens. I wouldn't want to prejudice you, but I think a lot of people here would tell you the same things. It's a pretty general feeling. You think Miss Joyce and Miss Biedel are charming, and they *are*—so long as you aren't a nurse and don't work for them."

Mrs. May rose from her chair and held out her hand.

"Well, what do you plan to do now?" asked Mrs. Wechsler as they shook hands.

"Oh, I'm going to rest till after the holidays, and then decide. Maybe I'll take private duty for a while," replied Mrs. May. "Anyway, I'll keep in touch with you."

"Do that," Mrs. Wechsler said, "and let's have lunch early in the new year and see how you are feeling then."

After Mrs. May had left, Mrs. Wechsler sat for some time pondering over the interview. Though she had no direct responsibility for the nursing service, she and Miss Joyce had worked informally together ever since Mrs. Wechsler joined the organization in 1945, a few months after Miss Joyce became the director of nursing. Now Mrs. Wechsler was wondering what sort of follow-up should be done on this interview, and what, if anything, she should talk over with Miss Joyce.

We have used this case with hundreds of people in a variety of hospital settings. On first reading, the dominant reaction is against Mrs. May because she is seen as "immature . . . pyschotic . . . a trouble-maker . . . a chronic complainer . . . frustrated . . . resenting authority . . . spoiled . . . demanding"; as a result, the discussants' solution is often "Let's get rid of her" or "Accept her resignation."

At this point the leader raises questions about specific complaints. Members often mention, with annoyance, that Mrs. May makes generalizations about nursing, old maids, other people's problems. It is important for you to help the group to sort out Mrs. May's angry denunciations and indictments. Take the coffee-break issue: Why should she and others have to have milk and crackers? Does the situation force her to "sneak" coffee year after year? How many of you prefer 10 A.M. milk to coffee? Could both be supplied? Is there any validity to her gripe?

Let's look at Mrs. May's OPD schedule. She states that 7:30 to 9 is used for reading the newspaper and gabbing and that no one reads the records. Since this is a waste of time as she sees it, she arrives late. On first impression, this tardiness seems to be flagrant rebellion. What are the factors which motivate her to break the rule? Since there is no mention of her *not* reading the cases and records, and since the Director of Nursing (Miss Joyce) says she is a good nurse, the implication is that Mrs. May gets her work done. If she prefers not to gab, what about the possibility of adjusting her schedule to permit her to report on duty later and leave later, or a reduced schedule if she is willing to have less take-home pay? Concern about establishing an undesirable precedent can be offset by the leader's pointing out that other nurses seem to enjoy that hour and a half to socialize "on company time."

We know that Mrs. May tried to talk to her supervisor about the OPD schedule. The reply was, "Miss Jason and Miss Perkins who preceded you were two of the best nurses we ever had, and they thought it important to be here at 7! Do you see why you shouldn't be?" Let's look at the human side of this supervisor's response. Isn't it true that most of us cringe when someone compares our accomplishment with that of someone who did it "better"? Our negative response perhaps is conditioned by early childhood experiences when teachers and other adults compared us to our sisters, brothers, or peers who were "shining lights." Being compared with the Misses Jason and Perkins is likely to make Mrs. May more resistant rather than to motivate her toward change. We may then ask: "Should the supervisor examine this 7:30 to 9 block to see how it is being used by the staff? Is Mrs. May's tardiness a symptom of the system?"

Also, Mrs. May angrily itemizes the shortcomings of the hospital. She criticizes the 15 months' to two years' backlog of patients waiting for admission to the surgical service. She ends by saying that because of the demands of Blue Cross and Blue Shield the "old fogies better watch their step." Immediately our "hackles" arise over her designation of colleagues as being old fogies. We see this as "unprofessional." Also we may identify ourselves with the nurses in that situation, and take the remark as a slur on all the nursing staff.

Our personal negative reactions divert our attention from the legitimacy of her criticism of the long waiting list and its serious effect on the life-saving goal of the hospital.

In this same outburst, Mrs. May accuses the supervisor of favoritism toward "Brownell." Does this, even if true, have anything to do with the closing of beds or with the shortage of nurses? Doesn't this undocumented accusation stir antagonism in us, and thus divert our attention from the real issue of the hospital's commitment to meeting the needs of the community?

What are some issues in the low glove count on Mrs. May's ward? How often has this happened? Where was the responsibility for the one low count—with Mrs. May, or the vacation replacement, or Mrs. Gerber? What is the value of Mrs. May's system of ordering gloves as compared to Mrs. Gerber's? Is there an established procedure?

On the issue of new-type splints, Mrs. May "jumped channels."

What motivated her to bypass the supervisor? Is better patient care any justification for a bypass? When a supervisor is ignored by her subordinates, should she ask herself, "Is it me as well as thee?"

We see that Mrs. May had an accumulation of gripes and concerns. She waited until her frustrations built up to the point at which they became threatening and explosive. She "blew-up" to the personnel director, who has no direct responsibility for nursing service. Mrs. May felt better, but is catharsis per se constructive in effecting change? When one is so angry and bitter, isn't she likely to drag in irrelevant and hearsay stories which cloud the major issues (e.g., her references to "nursing isn't a profession any more," relations between administration and other nurses, "old-maids," student shortage)? Were there nursing channels to handle grievances as they occurred? The Director, Miss Joyce, admits that she couldn't handle the situation. What help did *she* need? What about the accidental meeting with Mrs. Wechsler in the elevator? If Mrs. May is "a good nurse and one of our own graduates," is she worth saving?

There are many other issues to be analyzed in this case, as well as other ways of perceiving them. Who-can-do-what to bring about change? Is there a short-term and a long-term decision to be made? Since the purpose is to focus on supervisory processes, ask members to examine the situation from that point of view. Suggest that they assume the position of the supervised to test reactions.

6

CASES AND SITUATIONS

These cases and situations have been selected for use in early in-service sessions. It is hoped that finally the leader and group members will bring cases and situations from their own nursing areas for discussion.

Doris Owens' Special Treatment *

After 48 hours of severe pain in her right shoulder, unrelieved by home remedies, Doris Owens, a public health nurse, visited her physician on Thursday morning at about 10 o'clock. Dr. Wilson completed his examination and said in a kindly voice:

"Well, I would like you to go into University hospital." †

DORIS: You don't think it would just clear up if I applied heat at home and rested?

DR. WILSON: No, at this stage, I don't think so, and without treatment, it will tend to become worse.

* Permission was granted by the Board of Trustees of Boston University to reprint this case contained in *Case Studies in Nursing Service Administration,* Volume I, compiled by the faculty and graduate students of Boston University School of Nursing, and copyrighted 1954 by the Board of Trustees of Boston University. Copies of the case may be obtained through the Boston University Book Store (8/PBDOSTI). The assignment to group discussants is that of the authors.

† University Hospital was a teaching hospital, well known for its medical practice and its contributions to medical education and research.

DORIS: Well, I haven't slept for the past two nights and I can't stand it too much longer and keep on working.

DR. WILSON: There are two courses I can follow. I can inject it and give you immediate relief, which may be temporary. I would prefer to give you ACTH. We have had some rather dramatic results in cases such as yours by giving it slowly over a period of eight hours for four successive doses. This seems to be the type of case that has benefited. I think it would be worth trying. Can you do it?

DORIS: It will be difficult to arrange the time from my work. I *have* to be there late Friday afternoon and Saturday, during the middle of the day. If it means only four days, could the treatment be arranged so that I might leave the hospital for those periods? I would rather do something now than face a longer period of inactivity later.

A plan was evolved whereby treatment could be started at once and outside privileges arranged from 4:00 P.M. on Friday to 3:30 P.M. Saturday. By giving the fourth dose Sunday, it was hoped the condition would be relieved sufficiently to permit a return to work on Monday. The plan was as follows:

Admission to the hospital at once—Thursday 11:00 A.M.

Treatments	Tentative Hours
Thursday—8 hours	2–10 P.M.
Friday —8 hours	8 A.M.–4 P.M.
Saturday —8 hours	4–12 P.M.
Sunday —8 hours	9 A.M.–5 P.M.

Dr. Wilson appeared throughout the conversation to be giving consideration to Doris' physical discomfort, her future recovery, and her obligation to her work. At one point he said: "This is one of the times when the hospital should apply the policy of outside privileges to meet your needs, but probably this d— hospital won't be able to make the adjustment. It may also be difficult to secure a bed for you."

MISS HINES (his nurse-secretary): Oh, now, that is unfair, the hospital is overcrowded and they are doing the best they can.

Dr. Wilson laughingly agreed.

Miss Hines called the admitting office and after some discussion, a room was secured. Dr. Wilson called the resident, described the case and gave instructions about treatment, saying that the patient had to leave the hospital for an interval and that treatment should be planned around this absence.

Upon arrival on the ward at 11:15 A.M., Doris was greeted cordially by a staff nurse who escorted her to a room and assisted in getting her into bed. The head nurse, Miss Randall, came and inquired about her symptoms, asked if there was anything she would like and said that the doctor had been notified and would be there directly. She said Miss Hines had given her the plan of treatment and would call Doris' sister to notify her of Doris' decision to enter the hospital, since that had not been anticipated when she left home.

At 1:30 P.M., Miss Randall came again to say she had called the resident several times but was now unable to get any response. She was sure he would come before too long, however.

At 2:30 P.M., a technician took blood for examination. Doris was not only uncomfortable but was becoming restless and apprehensive about the long treatment which had been delayed so long that now it would extend into the night. The staff nurse and the head nurse made several visits, saying that there was always difficulty in getting experimental drugs. The pharmacy did not always have them and the research supply had to be secured by the resident. With increasing annoyance, Miss Randall finally announced: "If the resident doesn't get here soon, I am going to call Dr. Wilson to find out what to do."

Shortly after 3:00 P.M., she notified Dr. Wilson who said he would take care of it. At 3:30 P.M., a white-uniformed doctor came into the room, turned on the overhead light, placed some equipment on the dresser, and a tray with syringes and bottles on the overbed table. Finally Doris said, "Good afternoon," and received a barely audible response. The doctor continued to prepare equipment, looked at the patient's arm and asked her to remove her wristwatch. Miss Randall brought other equipment and was asked by the resident to mix the drug. She looked at him searchingly and confidently arranged the medication for him to mix * and left the room.

DORIS: I judge it is difficult to secure enough of this miracle drug.

RESIDENT: No, just some administrative confusion.

By 3:40 P.M., the intravenous was started and shortly after, the resident returned to take the patient's history and make a physical examination. To Doris, he showed little interest in her condition.

When supper was served, the aide made Doris comfortable so that with her free right hand, she fed herself. The head nurse and the evening nurse came in and looked at the intravenous apparatus frequently. The supervisor on her rounds observed that it was running. There

* It is a policy of the hospital that experimental drugs must be mixed by a physician.

were 1000 ml of fluid to be given. Because of the tediousness of remaining so quiet, Doris asked the evening nurse on one of her visits if it couldn't be speeded up. The nurse promptly made some adjustments in the flow of the fluid. Shortly before 10:00 P.M., Doris watched the last of the fluid disappear and called the nurse who removed the needle. Stiff and tired, Doris walked the length of the corridor to the bath. On return she was given a sedative which provided sufficient comfort, so she was wakened because of discomfort only twice during the night.

At 7:30 the next morning, a white-haired nurse, Miss Ray, aroused her with a cheerful good morning. The usual routines of temperature, breakfast, and bed-making during her bath were disposed of by the time the resident visited with his genial superior, the senior resident, who greeted Doris cordially with: "Good morning, I am Dr. Morris."

DORIS: Good morning, I don't think I have seen you before and I don't know this gentleman's name.

DR. MORRIS: Oh, Dr. Fernald. Well, have we succeeded in making you feel any more comfortable?

DORIS: It really is a little early to know.

Not to be put off today when time was of the essence, Doris reminded them that it was imperative that she be free by 4:00 P.M. The intravenous was started shortly after 9:00 A.M., this time, 500 ml. Miss Ray observed the intravenous frequently, always cheerful, chatting constantly and personally, and asking repeatedly what she might do. The head nurse adjusted the flow on two of several observations. Shortly after 4:00 P.M., Doris called to have the needle removed, and the second treatment was complete. The pain was less acute. Doris dressed and left the hospital.

Having been able to keep her appointments, Doris returned to the hospital the next day at 3:30 P.M., tired and uncomfortable from pain. By 4:30 P.M., the third intravenous of 500 ml was started. The resident had some difficulty in finding a vein and inserting the needle so that the bed was wet and soiled. There was no clamp in the tray to regulate the flow. The resident looked at the rate, left without speaking and did not return. A nursing student came later to check and, on being told the doctor had left it flowing at that rate, seemed to assume it was all right and did not adjust it. Following supper, Doris occupied herself with reading. After some three hours, she observed that only about 150 ml of the fluid remained and called the nurse who attached a clamp to slow the rate. The nurse then notified the doctor. By the time he arrived 10 minutes later, the needle had become clogged and had to be removed. After more probing for another vein, treatment was again started, with some uncertainty as to whether the vein was punctured. Within 15 to 20 minutes the surrounding tissues became swollen, causing considerable discomfort. Doris called a nurse who stated that it was obvious the fluid was flowing into the tissues and, because of the small amount remaining, removed the needle. Although nearly seven hours had elapsed since the treatment had been started, the actual time of administration was about four hours. Nervous and uncomfortable, Doris walked to the bath. On her return, the student urged that a back rub might be effective and gently applied lotion and powder, changed the soiled linen, and left her patient ready for sleep.

The next day, Sunday, Doris bathed while her bed was made and after some slight difficulty in which the bed was again badly soiled with blood and saline, the treatment was started by 10:30 A.M. Less frequent observations were made by the nurses, and toward the middle of the afternoon, Doris called attention to the fact that the flow appeared to have stopped. The nurse clamped it off and called the resident. Again, more probing was necessary, causing added discomfort before the needle was successfully inserted. The treatment was finally completed about 5:00 P.M.

In the afternoon Dr. Wilson visited the patient during the treatment.

After an evaluation of the results of these treatments, since little relief had resulted, he suggested that Doris should remain in the hospital for x-ray examination of the spine to determine the relationship between a developing arthritis and the present symptoms. Doris was a pretty despondent patient, in the still-soiled bed, when her sister, who had come to take her home, left her for another night in the hospital. During the night, in spite of a sedative, she wakened several times from discomfort. The only suggestion by the night nurse was the offer of another sedative. This she refused.

X-rays were taken in the middle of the next afternoon. Dr. Wilson then visited and decided on an injection of the bursa for the relief of the acute pain and another intravenous of ACTH. This was started at 9:30 P.M. Doris was given a sedative and settled for the night. The needle was inserted in the anterior surface of the arm on the affected side. Doris wakened shortly after 11:00 because of discomfort from position. By 12:45 P.M., the intravenous was completed. Doris called the night nurse who removed the needle, offered another sedative, which was refused, and left. After an hour of continued discomfort, Doris signalled again, stating that she believed if she could have "a good firm back rub," it might give some relief to her pain and tension, and she might get to sleep. The nurse, an uncommunicative young person, crisp in her uniform, appeared very confident. She gave a brisk, superficial rub for not more than a minute and was through. Doris turned, made herself as comfortable as possible and resigned herself to make the best of it. The night was long.

After conference with Dr. Wilson, Doris was discharged from the hospital late the next afternoon. The acute pain was somewhat relieved. Dr. Wilson advised physiotherapy twice a week temporarily and planned for further evaluation of her condition in a few weeks.

On return to her home and after time for reflection, Doris was considerably disturbed by her hospital experience. The confidence inspired by the kindness of the head nurse on her arrival had been sadly undermined by the delays, neglect, and uncertainties she had experienced during her stay. She felt that one could not fairly judge the effectiveness of the treatment, for it had not been skillfully administered nor according to plan, and little had been done to make her comfortable. The cost of the four days, exclusive of Dr. Wilson's fee, had been $127.00, of which $92.50 had been met by Blue Cross. Doris felt she had derived no real benefit. She wondered to whom she should talk about this experience which reflected so little credit on either the hospital or its personnel.

ASSIGNMENT TO GROUP DISCUSSANTS

Doris Owens finally decided to ask for an appointment with the Director of Nursing. After the conference, the Director of Nursing delegated the investigation of this nursing problem to the Head Nurse and Supervisor with a specific charge to come prepared with recommended action.

Assume the roles of the Head Nurse and Supervisor. Analyze the nursing care given to Doris Owens. Was she justified in her feelings? Give bases for your conclusions. What action should be recommended, if any? Who should carry out these recommended actions?

Mrs. Lindsay, Patient *

Mrs. Lindsay called her physician to visit her at home after four days of illness, during which time her condition had become increasingly acute. Dr. Bruce diagnosed her condition as acute gastroenteritis. He advised that she go to the hospital at once because of her weakened condition and dehydration, due to persistent vomiting. Dr. Bruce called the admitting office of the hospital and arranged for her admission to a semiprivate room in the Sherman Pavilion.

On arriving at the hospital, the taxi driver said: "You must mean the Grant House." Being unfamiliar with the hospital, Mrs. Lindsay and her sister, who accompanied her, left the taxi and entered Grant House. Mrs. Lindsay sat in a barren waiting room in an uncomfortable chair while her sister went to the reception desk and informed the receptionist that she had brought Mrs. Lindsay for whom Dr. Bruce had arranged admission.

It was 7:10 in the evening, and the receptionist appeared to have no knowledge of the patient's expected arrival. She called the admitting office which was located in another building, but received no answer. The call was repeated several times. Meanwhile, Mrs. Lindsay was becoming fatigued and appeared to her sister somewhat apprehensive. After waiting twenty minutes the receptionist finally received an answer from the clerk in the admitting office, with instructions to take the patient to a room in the next building.

A wheelchair was secured in which Mrs. Lindsay was taken to the floor where she was met by a graduate nurse, Miss Everett.

MISS EVERETT: Good evening, are you Dr. Ives' patient?

MRS. LINDSAY: No, Dr. Bruce is my physician.

MISS EVERETT: Oh, is he on the staff?

MRS. LINDSAY: I presume so. He made arrangements with the office for my coming here.

* Permission was granted by the Board of Trustees of Boston University to reprint this case contained in *Case Studies in Nursing Service Administration,* Volume I, compiled by the faculty and graduate students of Boston University School of Nursing, and copyrighted 1954 by the Board of Trustees of Boston University. Copies of the case may be obtained through the Boston University Book Store (18/SMLP1). The assignment to group discussants is that of the authors.

Miss Everett (to receptionist): She can go in private 341, the next to the last door on the left. I have to answer these lights.

Mrs. Lindsay's sister assisted her in getting into bed, unpacked her belongings, and, in observing their surroundings, became concerned that she was in a private rather than a semiprivate room. She reasoned, from her general knowledge of hospitals, that there were probably no more semiprivate rooms available.

Mrs. Lindsay complained of feeling too warm and her sister opened a window. The patient became restless and got her feet out from under the covers. After a time a student nurse entered the room.

Student (in a brusque tone): You will have to cover yourself or you will catch cold.

With no further consideration or identification she closed the window and left the room. A moment later a second student entered the room with a clothes book in which, with the assistance of the patient's sister, she listed her clothing. At the same time she secured a thermometer from the dresser and after shaking down the mercury placed it in Mrs. Lindsay's mouth and proceeded to count her pulse and respiration.

Within the next five minutes the clerk from the admitting office knocked and came into the room.

Clerk: I am sorry, but it is necessary for me to disturb you for some information. May I have your full name and residence? How old are you and what was the date of your birth? What is your present occupation? What was the occupation of your parents?

After a few more questions she said: "Would you kindly sign this?" handing a form to Mrs. Lindsay who signed it and seem agitated.

Mrs. Lindsay: I had expected a semiprivate room. It was my understanding that Dr. Bruce had made arrangements for it. I have Blue Cross insurance, but I do not feel that I can afford a private room.

Clerk: I know nothing about the Blue Cross arrangements nor of any arrangement having been made for a semiprivate room but I will look into the matter and see if there is one available.

Student: Well, I guess I won't go any further with this admitting procedure if she is going to be transferred.

The clerk and the nurse left. Thirty minutes went by without Mrs. Lindsay seeing anyone. She became restless. Since she understood Dr. Bruce had sent her to the hospital primarily for intravenous treatment to relieve her dehydration, she felt that it should have been started. Finally Miss Everett returned accompanied by a student nurse.

MISS EVERETT: We have been notified to transfer you to a semi-private room in the Sherman Pavilion.

Exhausted, irritated, and on the verge of tears, Mrs. Lindsay exclaimed: "A patient might die here before anyone paid any attention to how she felt."

MISS EVERETT: Oh it wouldn't happen if you were really sick.

She helped Mrs. Lindsay into her dressing gown, while her sister repacked her personal belongings. The student accompanied her to the Sherman Pavilion. After assisting her into bed, the student left and her sister again settled her, this time in a two-bed room which she shared with a white-haired woman. The other occupant was sitting up in bed surrounded with writing materials, boxes of cards, several vases of flowers, and a portable screen covered with greeting cards. She stopped her writing to observe the new patient and the activities in the room. No one spoke until the nurses had left the room. While Mrs. Lindsay's sister was arranging toilet articles, the patient said: "I am Jane Crowell. If you want anything, you will have to get that cord hanging over there. You may have to wait some time for there are not many nurses after 7 o'clock."

Mrs. Lindsay thanked her and began to toss about restlessly. Her sister attempted to fix her pillows and arrange the bedclothes for greater comfort.

MRS. LINDSAY: I feel very nauseated.

Her sister put on the signal light and found a basin in the table. Before a nurse answered, Dr Bruce arrived.

Dr. Bruce greeted Mrs. Lindsay in a friendly manner, drew the curtains between the patients, felt Mrs. Lindsay's pulse, and asked her how she felt. He stated that he was sorry about the confusion relating to her admission, and that he would leave orders which would soon be carried out and which he believed would make her more comfortable. Dr. Bruce left, followed shortly by her sister, and Mrs. Lindsay resigned herself to waiting.

Just before 11 P.M., a young resident physician entered the room with a tray containing mysterious bottles, tubing, instruments, and towels. Placing them on the table, he said, "I am Dr. Smith. I am just going to prick your arm and give you some fluid which I think will make you feel much better."

MRS. LINDSAY: Oh, I do hope so; I have waited so long. I am still nauseated and very warm and so tired. I have not slept much for four days.

Dr. Smith: Well, we will try to help that.

A nurse entered with a flask and a gravity pole. Dr. Smith took Mrs. Lindsay's arm to find a vein for the injection and, with no further conversation, inserted the needle and started the intravenous. After splinting the arm in a comfortable position, he turned to the nurse and muttered something under his breath, and before leaving, said, "For three hours, and you watch it." That had no real meaning to Mrs. Lindsay, but it was obvious that she must lie quietly. Having a mysterious fluid running into her vein was a little frightening. The nurse made no attempt to make Mrs. Lindsay comfortable and said nothing to reassure her in any way. She gave her a pill, looked at Jane Crowell in the next bed who was breathing noisily, turned out the light and left the room. Mrs. Lindsay closed her eyes with the feeling that something was being done for her at last. She finally dozed.

About 2 A.M. Mrs. Lindsay was aroused by a strange nurse who entered the room briskly but said in a quiet voice, "This is finished and I will remove all this so you can sleep." After finishing she said, "Is there anything you would like?" Mrs. Lindsay was drowsy and upon moving found herself stiff, so merely shook her head. She was given a sip of water and her pillows and bed made comfortable so that she dozed off shortly.

At about 5 A.M. Mrs. Lindsay was awakened by a strange nurse who entered her room rustling with starch, hair rather disheveled, a flashlight in one hand and thermometer in the other. With a crisp "good morning" to Mrs. Crowell, she drew back the curtains. Coming to Mrs. Lindsay's bed, she said, "Good morning, I hope you have slept enough to make you feel a little better." Mrs. Lindsay, feeling the night all too short, responded feebly that she guessed she had slept, but that her mouth was very dry and she felt hot and her stomach unsettled and sore. The nurse took her temperature and bustled from the room.

There was more or less continuous activity outside Mrs. Lindsay's room. Sometime later breakfast was served. Mrs. Crowell would have been talkative if encouraged, but Mrs. Lindsay was in no mood for it. During this time a boy came in the room and called: "Paper?"

Mrs. Lindsay: No thank you. (Aside) Oh, why do I have to be bothered with such things now?

MRS. CROWELL: That is a service the hospital provides. You may appreciate it tomorrow. I'll have one, Johnny.

Soon after Johnny left the room, a young man who stated that he was the hospital chaplain entered. To Mrs. Lindsay he appeared to lack composure and in response to his greeting she declared: "I don't feel like talking to anyone."

CHAPLAIN: I quite understand and will not disturb you now, but if at any time I can be of service, please call on me. (He left the room.)

Some time passed before a nurse came and said: "I'm going to fix you up now." She worked quickly and efficiently and made a few inconsequential pleasantries. During the process, to Mrs. Lindsay's surprise, she made her feel more comfortable than at any time since her admission to the hospital. The nurse was hardly finished before Dr. Smith returned to give her another intravenous. This ran for three hours. Nurses came and looked at it but did nothing. Mrs. Lindsay became restless and uncomfortable. Her signal cord was not within reach and she asked Mrs. Crowell, finally, as the fluid was nearly gone, if she would call a nurse. The needle was no more than removed when an aide came with a tray of liquids for her noon meal. It was placed so far from her reach that she did not bother with it. The aide returned shortly with a tray for Mrs. Crowell.

MRS. CROWELL: This food is so cold, how can anyone eat it? I would think they might have learned by this time that I can't eat cabbage.

AIDE. Well, I don't know anything about it. That is what I was told to bring you. (She turned abruptly and left the room.)

Mrs. Crowell ate listlessly portions of her lunch and when finished tossed her napkin toward the tray. It fell to the floor. No one came into the room until Mrs. Lindsay's sister came to see her an hour later. Unfinished trays remained at both patients' beds. Mrs. Lindsay appeared flushed, her bed in the disorder of a restless patient, and the room generally untidy. Mrs. Lindsay's sister found words of encouragement difficult in this atmosphere.

Mrs. Lindsay's treatment continued for three days, after which time her acute symptoms subsided; she began to take nourishment and to feel somewhat stronger. When Dr. Smith visited her, she asked him if she might go home. After examining her, he said it would depend on Dr. Bruce's judgment but that he would discuss it with him.

An hour before Mrs. Lindsay's sister's expected arrival the head nurse came in to tell her she could go home that day after Dr. Bruce's visit. This was the first time she had seen the head nurse. A nurse whom she assumed to be a supervisor had been in twice. Her interests appeared to be primarily with housekeeping and the care of flowers.

Dr. Bruce confirmed her discharge on his one o'clock visit and gave her instructions for the next few days and an appointment at his office.

When Mrs. Lindsay's sister arrived, she assisted her in dressing and again packed her personal belongings. A nurse came to see that she had everything and said that the nursing aide would discharge her. As she went by the head nurse's station, the head nurse said that she hoped she was going home feeling much better. At the same time the ward clerk handed her a stamped, self-addressed envelope saying the hospital would appreciate her filling out the enclosed questionnaire and returning it to them at her convenience.

A week later, at a morning conference, the hospital administrator gave Miss Gove, the Director of Nursing, three questionnaires, returned by patients, which he stated he thought she might wish to see and hoped she might be able to do something about. Two of them commented very favorably about the nursing care they had received. They were all signed and the third, written over Mrs. Lindsay's signature, was checked as follows:

QUESTIONNAIRE *

1. Were you received by the admitting and information personnel in a friendly ____ , formal _X_ , cold or abrupt ____ manner?
2. In general, do you feel that you received good ____ Average ____ , poor _X_ nursing care?
3. Did you feel that you were treated as an individual ____ , "just another case" _X_ , or as a machine without personal feelings ____ ?
4. In general, were you very pleased ____ , just satisfied ____ , disappointed _X_ ?

Miss Gove, the Director of Nursing, had been in her position only a short time, and this was her first experience as a Director. She was qualified by desirable academic preparation. The head nurse on the floor where Mrs. Lindsay had been a patient had been in her position for a year. She was young and had been given the appointment immediately on graduation from this hospital school. She was quite con-

* Questions relative to dietary and housekeeping service in this questionnaire have been omitted from this case as they appeared to be of little significance.

fident of her ability and rather lenient with her staff. The nurse in charge on this floor in the evening was an older nurse forced to work for personal reasons during this period. She had been in her position for several years and appeared to resent questioning. Miss Gove returned to her office debating in her own mind what she should do.

ASSIGNMENT TO GROUP DISCUSSANTS

(This case description is the result of an interview with Mrs. Lindsay's sister.)

Miss Gove, Director of Nursing, decided that both the evening and day supervisors should share the responsibility for follow-up on this situation.

We suggest that some members assume the roles of the evening and day supervisors to develop a plan for improved personnel performance.

Visiting in the Pediatric Unit *

For years all the head nurses and supervisors at Penn Hospital, a general hospital in a large eastern city, had met as a group every week for one hour on Tuesday afternoon. Shortly before Miss Mann † went there, however, head nurse meetings had been organized by administrative units. The pediatric head nurses and supervisor met with the neurological head nurses and supervisor since these services made up the Kent unit.

Following one of these Tuesday head nurse meetings Miss Rowe, pediatric supervisor, Miss James, head nurse, Ward 5, and Miss Mann returned to Ward 5, where Mrs. Duncan, ward secretary, left her desk and came over to speak with them as soon as they stepped off the elevator. Mrs. Duncan spoke hurriedly and nodded in the direction of a woman seated in the doctors' station.

MRS. DUNCAN: Mrs. Burns arrived on the floor at 1:30 P.M., the middle of rest hour, to see her son, Jimmy. I told her that she was mistaken about visiting hours; that our visiting hours were from 4:30 to 6:30 P.M. and that the children had a rest after lunch until 2:00 P.M. Mrs. Burns informed me that the visitor's desk had given her permission to come up and that she had been told visiting hours were unlimited . . .

MISS ROWE (interrupting): What?

MRS. DUNCAN: Yes, I called down to the desk and said a visitor had just informed me that she was allowed to come at anytime, but that I had not heard of any change in visiting hours from the 4:30 to 6:30 P.M. routine. The clerk read a memo from Dr. Newton [assistant director of hospital administration] dated two days ago, which stated that the pediatric visiting hours for ward service would be unlimited for parents and that the present hours, 4:30 to 6:30 P.M., for other

---

* Permission was granted by the Board of Trustees of Boston University to modify and reprint this case contained in *Case Studies in Nursing Service Administration,* Volume II, compiled by the faculty and graduate students of Boston University School of Nursing, and copyrighted 1954 by the Board of Trustees of Boston University. Copies of the unmodified case may be obtained through the Boston University Book Store (28/SBMVPU). The assignment to group discussants is that of the authors.
† A graduate student from a nearby university.

relatives and friends and the private service would remain unlimited.

MISS JAMES: Well, isn't that interesting!

MISS ROWE: I guess I will have to see Dr. Lord [chief of pediatric service] and find out what is going on, if I can!

Miss Rowe and Miss Mann went to Dr. Lord's office, but he was not there. Miss Rowe left word with his secretary that she would stop back later to see him.

The next morning when Miss Mann asked if Miss Rowe had seen Dr. Lord, she said she had seen him before going off duty. Dr. Lord told her that he and Dr. Newton had consulted together and arranged for the new visiting hours. He invited her and the head nurses to join the medical staff at a meeting to be held at 4:30 that afternoon, at which time he would announce to the group the change in hours. They could then discuss this problem as well as some of their medical problems.

When the group convened, Dr. Lord presented his change in policy with the explanation: "I feel the department is lagging behind the progressive trends of the time. The emphasis on psychological needs, as a part of total medical care is not a new concept. Yet I feel the department is violating this concept by continuing such a rigid regime of visiting hours for children. Therefore, I wish to see us adopt unlimited visiting hours."

The majority of the medical house staff were vehemently opposed to this change. The discussion was lively and heated and dominated by the opposition group. They felt they had very little time now to see patients, and if parents were going to be around all the time, they would never be able to find enough time to complete their work. They also felt they were being lenient enough by permitting those parents who were not able to come in at regular hours to make special arrangements for more convenient visiting hours.

The nursing group had held a discussion of the nurse's role in relation to parents and their children at a previous head nurse meeting. The subject came about when Miss Black, head nurse, Ward 6, made a complaint about the frequent interruptions she encountered throughout the day because parents were allowed unlimited visiting privileges on the private pediatric floor. Miss Lang, the director of nursing service, who officiated at the head nurse meeting in Kent unit, in the absence of an assistant director, recognized the need for a discussion of the topic and devoted the entire meeting to it. There was a free exchange of ideas, but no agreement among the group was reached at this one session. The decision was made to continue the discussion the following week. Unfortunately, at the next head nurse meeting Miss Lang had other business on the agenda to discuss with the group, so that there was no opportunity to resume the previous week's topic. The subject was dismissed and forgotten in the weeks that followed.

Therefore, when the nurses attended this joint medical and nursing conference, the nurses did not actively participate in the discussion. They mentioned their willingness to try out any suggestion, to prove or disprove its worth, upon which the group as a whole might decide. By the end of the conference, however, the group had not reached any concrete decision. The pediatric nursing staff was not notified of any further group discussion on this policy change.

Six weeks passed during which time very few parents of the ward patients came in any earlier than 2:30 or 3:30 P.M., and these were a minority. Miss Mann inquired of the two head nurses on the ward service if they had found the unrestricted visiting hours disrupting.

MISS JAMES: There has been no official notification sent around concerning the change. Most parents still come in at the usual hours and a few have made special arrangements with the doctors to come in at a more convenient time for them. I do not think we have been following the new directive literally.

MISS STANLEY: There has been no noticeable change in the pattern of the majority of visitors on my ward.

Later that day Miss Mann asked Miss Rowe how she thought the unrestricted visiting hours had been working.

MISS ROWE: It will be interesting for you to read this memo I just received from Dr. Bellin, the pediatric resident. It is the first notification we have had since we met with the house staff and Dr. Lord.

Miss Mann read the new visiting hour policy which appeared to her to be almost identical to the policy that had previously been in effect. The old policy allowed parents to visit between 4:30 to 6:30 P.M. daily, unless this time was inconvenient for them. In such cases, special arrangements were made upon a request to the doctor in charge of the child's care. The doctor wrote or gave a verbal order of the special hours for that particular parent to the head nurse who, in turn, notified the visitor's desk in the lobby of the hospital. Relatives and friends were allowed to come to the floor one at a time during the regular visiting hours, and no children under sixteen years of age were allowed to visit. The new policy stated that individual arrangements would be made between the parents and the doctor at the time of admission of their child, for the hours most convenient for them to visit. The doctor would write an order in the doctor's order book to that effect, so the nursing staff would know when to expect the parents. Visitors, other than the immediate family, might come one at a time and only between the hours of 4:30 to 6:30 P.M. weekdays and 2 to 3.30 P.M. on Sunday. No children under sixteen years of age would be allowed to visit because of the danger of spreading communicable disease.

MISS ROWE: I have not taken this notice up with the head nurses yet. I intend to do so the first of next week. We haven't been anxious to start more frequent visiting while the floors have been in the process of being redecorated anyhow. So I don't think the nurses or the doctors have informed the parents about unlimited visiting as Dr. Lord proposed several weeks ago. I know the doctors objected strenuously to the idea at the meeting we had, so I guess they have worked on Dr. Bellin in the meantime to keep control of visiting hours in their hands.

A day or two later while Miss Mann was having a conference with the director of nursing service, Miss Lang, she inquired: "Would you tell me if you were approached by Dr. Lord and Dr. Newton in relation to the proposed change in visiting hours for the pediatric service?"

MISS LANG: No, I was not. I learned of the new policy through Miss Rowe. I was disturbed by the manner in which Dr. Newton had handled it, but I took the line of passive resistance and did not go to him and argue out my views. However, I shall not forget this incident and the next time a proposal for a radical change comes up, I intend to use this incident as an example. Getting acceptance of unlimited visiting hours was doomed from the beginning because no one was prepared for it.

MISS MANN: I felt that the nursing staff would have been willing to give it a fair trial. True they were skeptical, but I thought they were open minded.

MISS LANG: Did you attend the head nurse meeting when Miss Black started a discussion on her problem with parents? She told how often she was interrupted, so that it made it impossible for her to complete her work within an eight-hour period.

MISS MANN: No, I was not present at that meeting, but I heard about it from Miss Rowe. I attended the meeting the following week because I was interested in hearing the continuation of that discussion, but unfortunately other business took up the hour so the group did not get an opportunity to resume the topic.

MISS LANG (rising and indicating the conference was over): The arguments of the girls convinced me that they had no insight into their role in relation to parents, and the responsibility they should assume when families were visiting. I don't think my nursing staff was any more ready to accept unlimited visiting than the doctors.

As Miss Mann left Miss Lang's office, she wondered what had been accomplished and what she would do about this if she were in Miss Lang's place. What kind of preparation would sell such a change to the staff?

ASSIGNMENT TO GROUP DISCUSSANTS

Miss Lang has decided that the best way "to sell such a change" is to delegate the job to Miss Rowe, Supervisor. Analyze the case and test alternate solutions from the point of view of Miss Rowe.

Consider also the principles and problems of instituting change and meeting resistance to change which a supervisor encounters in other areas. Refer to specific *change* attempts from your own experience.

Manchester Hospital *

Manchester Hospital was a general hospital of 100 beds located in a suburban area of a large city. Mrs. Penn, the director of nursing, had been in her position approximately eight years, and during the war had employed Joan Whittimore as her assistant. At that time Mrs. Penn had been glad to relinquish some of her responsibilities for staffing to Miss Whittimore. At the end of five years in her position, Joan was well aware that her idea of maintaining a stable staff by providing each unit with three to four hours of nursing care per patient per day was contrary to Mrs. Penn's idea of staffing, which was to move graduate and student nurses from one unit to another as needed throughout the day. Joan was also aware that Mrs. Penn felt more money was spent on nursing service than was necessary. Not that Mr. Stone, the hospital administrator, had commented, for since Mrs. Penn had complained that he had interfered in her work, he had allowed her to proceed as she saw fit.

Today Joan Whittimore looked with exasperation into the empty office of Mrs. Penn. This was the fifth time that day that she had visited the director's office, in the hope of seeing her, to no avail. It was now near the supper hour, and it appeared that Mrs. Penn had left her office until the following day.

Joan hesitated in the doorway of the office for a moment, then, walking over to the desk, she dialed the telephone operator and asked to be connected with Mrs. Penn's apartment.

When Mrs. Penn answered, Miss Whittimore said somewhat testily: "Mrs. Penn? I've been trying to reach you all day to find out what to do about Miss Parke. If she's going to take over when Miss Howe leaves Ward A, she ought to spend some time there before Miss Howe goes. She doesn't know the ward. It's now Monday night and Miss Howe leaves on Saturday."

* Permission was granted by the Board of Trustees of Boston University to reprint this case contained in *Case Studies in Nursing Service Administration,* Volume I, compiled by the faculty and graduate students of Boston University School of Nursing, and copyrighted 1954 by the Board of Trustees of Boston University. Copies of the case may be obtained through the Boston University Book Store. (22/SFOMH). The assignment to group discussants is that of the authors.

"I don't want Miss Parke to go to Ward A until after Miss Howe leaves," Mrs. Penn replied.

"But why?" queried Miss Whittimore.

"Because I don't," answered Mrs. Penn emphatically. "I don't want Miss Parke to have anything to do with Miss Howe."

"But," objected Miss Whittimore, "there's a lot of difference between Ward A and Ward C where Miss Parke has been working. You know that Ward A is the hardest ward in the house. And Miss Parke has not done any head nursing here."

"Well, I don't want her to go to Ward A until Miss Howe is out of the house," Mrs. Penn reiterated.

"I don't know who can tell her about the ward when she gets there, then. I simply can't spend three or four weeks with her and carry my other work, too. I did it when Miss Trude came, and I spent a month trying to break in Bill. But I simply can't do it again. I've got too much to do," was Miss Whittimore's response.

"You won't have to," replied Mrs. Penn in an even tone of voice. And then, her voice rising, she continued, "I've had just about all of this that I intend to take. You are into everything—making arrangements that I know nothing about. I don't know half of the things that are going on around here."

Miss Whittimore's sharp intake of breath was plainly heard. After a momentary pause, she responded in a somewhat conciliatory tone:

"What you are saying may be true. I may be doing a great many things that you don't know about. But if I'm doing things that you think I ought not to, I don't know which things they are. Time after time, I try to find you to talk something over, but you are either too busy to see me or not here. This is the fifth trip I've made to your office today to ask you about Miss Parke. Now, if I am doing things which you don't want me to do, then you're the one who has to say which things they are." Miss Whittimore ended her comments on a note of finality.

Mrs. Penn was silent following Miss Whittimore's reply, and then, in a voice which seemed less tense, inquired: "What arrangements have you made about the operating room? What did you tell Miss Wessel? I don't know what you've done."

"I haven't made any arrangements in the operating room," Miss Whittimore replied. "I spoke to Miss Maynard and asked her what she thought about taking over the administration when Miss Green leaves. Then I asked Miss Wessel if she would be interested in taking over the teaching up there. I simply asked them what we had discussed beforehand, and I told you what they said at the time. That must be all of three or four weeks ago."

"And you haven't done anything more since?" asked Mrs. Penn.

"No, I haven't," Miss Whittimore replied.

The conversation continued for a few seconds more, ending upon Mrs. Penn's: "Well, we'll see."

Two weeks later, Miss Whittimore stopped in the workroom of the operating room as she was making her morning rounds. Ruth Maynard and Sylvia Wessel were standing at the worktable, examining the joints of hemostats.

Norma Green, who had been the operating room supervisor for seven years, had been gone a week. She had given her resignation a month prior to her leaving. Her approaching marriage had provided the hospital with a fair amount of excitement because most of the nursing staff was to be invited to her wedding reception.

The nurses' assignment sheet hanging on the bulletin board was in Ruth Maynard's handwriting. She had been Norma's assistant for four years. The two not only worked well together but were close personal friends and roommates. Norma had given over the scheduling of rooms and the assigning of nurses to Ruth, thinking that some administrative detail would interest her. Ruth was a somewhat "high-strung" girl, exceptionally quick in her movements but inclined to moodiness. She often became impatient and even tearful with new personnel because they were slow or showed little aptitude for operating room work.

Ruth looked up from her instruments and in her usual rapid manner of speaking asked: "Do you know what we're supposed to be doing up here? Mrs. Penn told me over the telephone a week ago that I was to take over the administration of this place and Sylvia was to teach the students—we were to have a meeting the next day to talk over our duties. That's the way they do things around here. Always wait until the last minute. You're supposed to carry on and guess what they mean."

Miss Whittimore motioned the two girls into an adjoining workroom which was empty. Closing the door behind her, she said, "I'm in the same situation myself. I don't know what I'm supposed to be doing either. I'm not going to try to settle this because I'm not getting myself involved with any of the graduates. Why don't the two of you go to Mrs. Penn and say that you want it straightened out?"

"I'm not going," Ruth said. "After all, it's their hospital. If they don't care what's going on, I don't see why I should. It isn't as if they hadn't known Norma was leaving. She's been having all the others down to talk to them."

"Having who down—what are you talking about?"

"Having Jean and Esther and the rest of them."

"What's she talking about to them?"

"Oh, she wants to know if they get along up here and who they think would make a good supervisor. They come up and tell me. . . ."

"Oh, for goodness sakes," Miss Whittimore said, "she ought to know you two by now. Well, I don't know. It seems to me that you could decide between yourselves which things you are going to do. You both know what has to be done. Can't you list them and then decide who'll do what? You're on good terms now, but if you keep getting into each other's way, you'll end up mad at each other. The first thing you know, the girls will begin to take sides. Believe me, my young ladies, if you get a split started up here in the staff, it will be a sorry day, because it takes years to stop a thing like that once it's started."

"What are you doing?" Sylvia asked. "Aren't you supervising?"

"No, I'm going around, keeping myself busy, but I'm not having anything to do with the graduates," Miss Whittimore replied.

"Who's attending to things?" Sylvia inquired.

"I'm referring everything to Mrs. Penn. I guess she must be," Joan replied.

"What does Mr. Stone think about it?"

"I don't know," replied Miss Whittimore. "I simply told him that I would not do any of my former work because Mrs. Penn felt I was overstepping. I thought he should know that I wasn't doing the work I had been doing. Well, I'll go along. . . ."

Three weeks later, Miss Whittimore stopped at the desk in the operating room to examine the students' experience records. "How are things?" she asked Miss Wessel.

"All right," said Miss Wessel, "only I can't be teaching or supervising students if I'm tied up running a room. That Dr. Osborne! If I as much as glance out the door, he begins to fuss that the light isn't just right, or the silk is too fine, or it's too noisy. I don't know of anyone who makes any more noise than he does out at the scrub sink."

Miss Whittimore looked a bit doubtful. "I don't know that we can have two people not assigned to rooms. It may not be possible."

"I don't mean when it's busy," Sylvia replied. "But a day or so when the students first come isn't enough time for teaching."

Miss Whittimore stopped to speak to Miss Maynard:

"How are you doing?"

"O.K." Ruth answered. "Busy."

"Have you seen Mrs. Penn yet?"

"No."

"I was wondering if you had to assign Sylvia to run a room?"

"I have to," Miss Maynard replied with emphasis. "We wouldn't have enough nurses to circulate. I run rooms myself."

"I know that," Miss Whittimore said, "but, on the other hand, there isn't too much point in having someone to teach and supervise the students if she can't get to them."

"I suppose there isn't," Ruth answered, "but I don't know what we can do about it. I never assign her on the days the new students come."

"Do you think you could give her the short cases? If you have to put her in a long case, try to put her where the students are scrubbed for the first time."

"Well, I'll try. Can't promise anything, though," Ruth responded.

Miss Whittimore left the operating room wondering what more she could do.

SUGGESTION TO GROUP DISCUSSANTS

In the analysis of this case be sure to include diagnosis of the supervisory processes in the relationship between the director of nursing and her assistant even though neither has the position of supervisor.

Brattle Hospital—Clinic *

Mr. Smith had been a head nurse on the male convalescent ward in Brattle Hospital for the past two years. The eighteen patients on his floor were diverse in diagnosis, including psychoneurosis, psychosis, and senility. Their ages ranged from the early thirties to the late seventies. Female patients also lived on this ward for the therapeutic value which the physicians felt was gained from association with the opposite sex.

There were usually four students assigned to this unit—two affiliating students and two Brattle Hospital junior students. The rotation of the affiliating and basic students was staggered. Their educational program was somewhat different due to their year in the school. Mr. Smith said that because of the scarcity of help and the students' educational differences, he could not include all the students at one time in his clinics, thus, he divided them into two groups—one for the affiliates and one for the basic junior students.

Recently, it was reported that the junior students assigned to his ward complained to the assistant director of the school, Mrs. Mann, that Mr. Smith was discriminating against them by not including them in the clinics with the affiliates, and that he wasn't giving them any clinical instruction.

On Monday morning of the last week in April, following her receipt of the student's complaint, Mrs. Mann went to the ward about eight o'clock accompanied by Mr. Hamilton, Supervisor and Clinical Instructor on the Male Service. When they arrived, Mr. Smith was giving a clinic, to the one affiliate student on duty, in the card room.

MRS. MANN (without preamble to the student): You'll have to leave now, I have some business to discuss with Mr. Smith. . . . The students complained to me about your being partial to the affiliates and here I find you with one affiliate and the juniors out on the ward. You

---

* Permission was granted by the Board of Trustees of Boston University to reprint this case contained in *Case Studies in Nursing Service Administration,* Volume II, compiled by the faculty and graduate students of Boston University School of Nursing, and copyrighted 1954 by the Board of Trustees of Boston University. Copies of the case may be obtained through the Boston University Book Store (38/SCRBHC). The assignment to group discussants is that of the authors.

know the juniors are students too, and you owe it to them to include them in the clinics, if only because they're our own students.

MR. SMITH: You know this is the affiliates' last week here on the ward. Mrs. Thomas, my assistant, is on vacation and I'm behind on their clinics. I'm trying to catch up to give them all I usually cover in the course of a month.

MRS. MANN: There's no reason to give them individually. You should give them together for they can help each other to understand the material.

MR. SMITH: If I give them together early in the morning, I wouldn't have anyone on the ward. I don't feel I can leave an attendant alone on the ward at this time.

MRS. MANN: The other wards are able to give them in the morning, and there's no reason why you can't do it on a ward like this.

MR. SMITH: I still don't think I can because there are medicines to give, patients to get up, and patients who need support early in the morning.

MRS. MANN: If you didn't waste so much time running around and at the canteen, you'd have time to give clinics.

MR. SMITH (apparently upset): I don't go there more than twice a month at the most and probably less than anyone else in the hospital. It doesn't seem logical that after two years of teaching without complaints you'd barge in and make these complaints in this manner. We don't get any recognition or praise anyway for what we do and I feel that I could stand some help on how to give clinics so that I can do a better job.

MRS. MANN: I know, Joe, that you are capable of doing a good job. The students have all liked your clinics in the past. You have done a good job, Joe. You have a lot of ability and good judgment. Keep up the good work. One other thing, I wish you'd get on the ball with your ward reports. They are coming in late, long after the student leaves the ward. If they're to be helpful they should be done before the student leaves the ward.

MR. SMITH: Yes, I know I am lax, but I'll try to do better. When I fall down, will you remind me?

MRS. MANN (smiling): All right. Don't worry, we'll remind you.

MR. HAMILTON: Perhaps I'm partly to blame for this because I can't get around enough to check on them.

MR. SMITH: Even though you do check, I'm still somewhat lax, but it helps to keep me reminded.

MRS. MANN: I'm sorry to have bothered you, and I'm sure you'll get along all right.

As they walked to the door, Mrs. Mann shifted the conversation to questions about his patients.

They left the ward about nine o'clock as Mrs. Thomas came on duty. She was just returning from her vacation.

MR. SMITH: Come in. I'm mad. I'd like to tell you what just happened. Mrs. Mann just bawled me out. She told me the students complained about the way I was giving the clinics—I was discriminating against them. Since she also accused me of wasting time in the canteen, I'm going down and waste some. . . . Here, I'd better give you a report on the patients before I go.

MRS. THOMAS: This whole thing doesn't sound right, and I don't know why juniors should complain. (She picked up the students' folders.) They haven't even recorded the clinics you've given, except this one student.

MR. SMITH: That's right. You know, I think I'll keep a record myself of everything I give the students, formal and informal, and she can check it against what the students say they get. I guess I'll go waste some of the time she says I do.

Later that morning, Mr. Smith met Mr. Hamilton.

MR. SMITH: You know, I didn't like that business this morning at all. Mrs. Mann should have called me either to your office or hers without coming to the ward. It's the same old story, when you do things right, you never hear anything, but when something goes wrong they jump all over you. I still don't think I can give the clinics jointly because of the difference in the students.

MR. HAMILTON: I know how you feel. I didn't like it either. I agree with you that you can give better clinics to them separately.

ASSIGNMENT TO GROUP DISCUSSANTS

Assume the role of the supervisor. Mr. Smith has come to you with the above story. What are the issues and how would you handle the situation? What needs to be known about techniques of group teaching as contrasted to one-to-one teaching?

Mrs. Senn, Staff Nurse *

Miss James was the head nurse on a 25-bed general pediatric ward for children between the ages of 6 and 18 years. Not only did the ward have a rapid turnover of patients and a full census throughout most of the year, but it was also a teaching unit for internes and resident doctors, for the hospital's nursing students, and for other students from affiliating schools of nursing.

Whenever she thought about the staffing situation on many of the other services in the hospital, Miss James felt fortunate to have her ward staffed as well as it was. She had an excellent assistant head nurse, two full-time staff nurses, one part-time staff nurse for three days a week, and an efficient nurse's aide, as well as the nursing students who were assigned in varying numbers according to their rotation.

One of her staff nurses, Mrs. Senn, was giving her some concern, however. Mrs. Senn had been employed about five months earlier. She had been working on Miss James' ward for this entire period, but she had appeared to have a difficult time adjusting and was still not accomplishing the amount of work or giving the kind of nursing care that Miss James expected of her graduates. Miss James found Mrs. Senn difficult to understand and to handle in many situations. She appeared insecure and defensive and on many occasions attempted to cover up her feelings with excessive chatter. After Mrs. Senn had been at work six weeks, Miss James had a conference with her in order to offer constructive criticism and guidance. She asked Mrs. Senn if she would try to concentrate on organizing her work better, so that she could carry a heavier assignment, and if she would please follow the procedures set up in this hospital, instead of those she had learned in her own school. During this conference and on several subsequent occasions Mrs. Senn offered the excuse that her way "was easier" for

---

* Permission was granted by the Board of Trustees of Boston University to reprint this case contained in *Case Studies in Nursing Service Administration,* Volume II, compiled by the faculty and graduate students of Boston University School of Nursing, and copyrighted 1954 by the Board of Trustees of Boston University. Copies of the case may be obtained through the Boston University Book Store (29/SBMMSSN). The assignment to group discussants is that of the authors.

her, or "seemed more efficient." Each time Miss James pointed out that uniformity of procedures was important when there were students to be taught. Not only did the students learn from their clinical instructor, but also by their observation of the graduate staff's techniques. Mrs. Senn did not seem to grasp the necessity of conforming, however. Now, just this past weekend, Mrs. Senn had encountered more difficulty on two occasions—one, in her relationship with a patient, and the other with a parent of one of the patients. Miss James decided she must discuss the situation with Miss Rowe, her supervisor, when she came on rounds.

When Miss Rowe arrived on the ward, she was greeted by Miss James—"Good morning, did you have a nice weekend?"

Miss Rowe: Yes, thank you. I didn't do anything exciting, however. Do you have any special problems you need me for, before I see the patients?

Miss James: Yes. My problem is Mrs. Senn. Once again, she got into difficulty on two different occasions over the weekend, because of her behavior.

Miss Rowe: Just what happened?

Miss James: She was assigned to Bobby, an eleven-year-old ulcerative colitis patient, on Saturday morning. She handled him very poorly. I overheard the following conversation as breakfast trays were being served:

Mrs. Senn: Here's your breakfast, Bobby (as she placed his tray in front of him on his bed).

Bobby: I hate eggs cooked that way. I won't eat them.

Mrs. Senn: You'll just have to eat them that way or go hungry.

Bobby: Well, I won't!

Miss James: Mrs. Senn left the room then and continued passing trays. I probably should have spoken to her then and there, but at the moment, I decided to ignore it until Mrs. Senn was in a better mood. Later in the morning I was going around the ward and I went into Bobby's room to check on everything and I found him crying. I asked him what the matter was. It took several minutes for him to quiet down and tell me that Mrs. Senn was "mean"—she "picked" on him. I asked him why he felt that she did. He replied that she had been cross because he hadn't stopped working on his belt immediately when she was ready to give him his bath. Mrs. Senn had just taken the leather and tools out of his hands. I did my best to smooth things over, but Bobby had to get in the last word by saying he did not want her for his nurse again.

MISS ROWE: Saturday must have been one of Mrs. Senn's bad-mood days.

MISS JAMES: Sunday the second episode occurred. Mrs. Senn was working 3 to 11:30 P.M. Mrs. Hunter was still visiting her daughter, Betty, at 7:30 P.M. Mrs. Senn went into the room and told Mrs. Hunter she had overstayed visiting hours by one hour already, so she would have to leave. Mrs. Hunter tried to explain that she had permission from Dr. Rand to remain until 8:00 P.M. Mrs. Senn said that she hadn't been informed that any exception was made and asked Mrs. Hunter to leave immediately. Mrs. Hunter left but was very upset—so upset as a matter of fact, that she called Dr. Rand after she arrived home.

Dr. Rand called Mrs. Senn and me together the first thing this morning. He apologized for not having passed the word along about the permission for extending the visiting hours, but he said that that did not excuse Mrs. Senn for the manner in which she had handled the situation. He said he had been right on the floor that evening, so Mrs. Senn could have come to him and checked with him if she had only stopped and thought.

Mrs. Senn also apologized and admitted she had been hasty and too abrupt, but said so many of the parents tried to get away with things that she had only tried to enforce the rules. Dr. Rand said that was her duty, but there was a tactful way of doing it, and that was that.

MISS ROWE: Well, it looks as if we'd better get together and discuss what we are going to do about Mrs. Senn. You have to get back to doctors' rounds, so I will see you later and we can set a time.

MISS JAMES: That will be fine.

As Miss Rowe walked down the corridor, she recalled a conversation with Mrs. Senn a few days after her assignment to work on Miss James' ward, when she had told Miss Rowe that her husband was Japanese and that they had come here in order that he might do graduate work at a nearby university. Though Miss Rowe was temporarily surprised, she asked in what field he was studying and was told that he was studying electrical engineering. Mrs. Senn was also taking one evening course in another university. Mr. Senn wished to work part time while studying to help out financially but had had difficulty in finding the kind of work he wanted.

Because of days off and of the pressing routine duties, it was Friday of the same week before Miss Rowe and Miss James could get together. They met in the conference room off Miss James' ward.

MISS ROWE: How long ago did you have your last conference with Mrs. Senn?

MISS JAMES: It was just after the holidays—about six weeks ago. The doctors had come to me with a complaint. It would appear that Mrs. Senn says things without thinking. For example: she said to Johnnie when he asked if he could get up, that if she had the "say" she would let him up. Another time Paul objected to taking his medication and Mrs. Senn said—if it were only up to her, he would not be getting it. The children have repeated these things to the doctors which has made them furious. About three weeks prior to that conference I talked with her also because she had not adjusted to the ward in the six weeks since she had come to pediatrics. Mrs. Senn has now shown some improvement. She now complies with most of our procedures; she is less talkative. However, she still does not work fast enough nor organize her work efficiently. At times, she is still very tactless.

MISS ROWE: It seems as though another conference with Mrs. Senn is necessary. If she shows no improvement nor desire to be helped by you, then I think I had better step in and have a chat with her and tell her she is on probation and must show improvement or else. Do you think you have enough concrete evidence to support your statements, Miss James?

MISS JAMES: Yes, I have a page of anecdotes, so I feel prepared for another interview with her. I will try and see Mrs. Senn this afternoon or tomorrow and let you know what she has to say.

The next day Miss James reported the results of her interview with Mrs. Senn to Miss Rowe. She said she felt Mrs. Senn was very much on the defensive all through the interview. Miss James commented first about her difficulty in adjusting and her inability to carry a patient assignment that Miss James considered suitable for a graduate nurse. Mrs. Senn replied that she just couldn't seem to get finished as quickly as she used to in the past. She complained of being tired and felt that she had to work split hours too often. Mrs. Senn said that she often went to bed at 8:30 P.M. during the week in order to keep going. Miss James told her that she was doing only her share of split time and that it was impossible to make it any less frequent than two times a week and the occasional three times, because then it would be unfair to the other staff members. Mrs. Senn recognized that fact but still wished something could be done for all of them.

Miss James said she commented also on the fact that she noticed that at times Mrs. Senn was not as patient with the children as she might be. Mrs. Senn replied that she was aware that she said things sometimes in such a way that people took offense and that she had been trying to be more careful; but again it happened mostly when she was so tired she could hardly keep going. Mrs. Senn said she was also upset by the fact that she and her husband were trying to make ends meet on her salary. He had not been able to find the kind of work he wanted to do and so was now going to take anything in order to tide them over until he could locate the type of job he wanted. Miss James said she could understand that this situation was quite a burden and responsibility for her and asked if there was anything she could do to help Mrs. Senn out in any way. Mrs. Senn said that no, there wasn't.

At the close of the interview Miss James decided that she would wait and see if the conference had any results by noting any change in Mrs. Senn in the next few weeks.

A few days later a field student, Miss Mann, who was working in the hospital, was talking with Mrs. Senn about the over-all orientation program given to new graduates employed at this hospital. Miss Mann and Mrs. Senn had met in an evening course in which they were both enrolled at one of the local universities. Mrs. Senn was in the treatment room where she was cleaning and straightening up equipment.

MISS MANN: I missed you in class the last few weeks of the semester. Were you ill or did you decide to drop out of the course?

MRS. SENN: I had to drop out. I found I just couldn't do it. I wasn't able to keep up with the work, carry a full-time job, and keep house.

MISS MANN: That is quite a load to attempt.

MRS. SENN: Yes, but I used to be able to do it, before I came up here. I went to school three nights a week, worked, and managed the apartment. I don't know what has changed me so—I have kind of lost interest in school now for one thing. Another thing—everyone and everything seems to be a lot different here in Philadelphia compared to Kansas where we used to live. People are so stuffy and cocky. You would think no other place in the United States had as good hospitals as there are here. They brag about the —— Clinic. I never heard of it before I came here. I have worked in many different hospitals, but I never came up against the conservatism you find around here.

MISS MANN: We Philadelphians have always had a reputation of being reserved.

MRS. SENN: Well, I certainly have found them mighty cool.

MISS MANN: Can you remember back to the first few weeks here in the hospital? I am interested in what you were given in your orientation to nursing in this hospital.

MRS. SENN: I remember I spent the whole first morning with Miss Hood, the supervisor in charge of the orientation program. I heard a brief history of the growth and development of this hospital, the organizational structure of the nursing service as it functions now, and I was taken on a tour of the hospital. Then in the afternoon, I reported to this floor and was oriented to the ward and introduced to the patients. The second day I came on duty here in the morning and had an assignment. In the afternoon I spent a couple of hours with Miss Hood again. She went over medications and the metric system and some of the special equipment with which I was not familiar, such as chest suction, gastric suction, and the intravenous sets they use and some of the oxygen equipment. That was about all.

MISS MANN: You had no further classes with Miss Hood, then?

MRS. SENN: No, I just saw her those two times.

MISS MANN: What about your introduction to pediatrics?

MRS. SENN: I have gone to a few student classes on procedures but mostly I have learned on the job.

Later Miss Mann talked with Miss James about the orientation of new staff nurses. Miss James said that she had no plan for a formal orientation. The new graduates were taught pediatric procedures by the educational supervisor with a student group. If the new graduate could not attend these classes, she was instructed individually as she met each new procedure. Her patient load was scaled according to difficulty, just as Miss James planned for the students, except that she expected the new graduate to adjust more quickly. She and her assistant gradually taught the new nurse the clerical work and routine charge duties she needed to know. They saw that she was oriented to evening duties and night duties before being assigned to work those shifts. There was no set pattern nor any program outlined on paper. Miss James said they did not know what material was covered by Miss Hood in the first week's orientation to the hospital unless they asked the new graduate herself.

ASSIGNMENT TO GROUP DISCUSSANTS

What are the supervisory problems with which the head nurse or supervisor should be concerned? What plan of action would you take? Consider alternative plans.

Miss Connor Resigns *

While Miss Rowe was on her week's vacation, Miss Paulson, the other supervisor in the Kent unit on the neurological service covered the pediatric floors. Miss Rowe was two days late returning from vacation because of illness. The two supervisors met following the regular joint Wednesday morning conference, and Miss Rowe was briefed about the happenings of the previous week.

Among other things Miss Rowe learned that a second episode concerning the Koch sisters' time off had ensued, and that Miss Connor, a pediatric staff nurse, had submitted her resignation the day Miss Rowe went on vacation, to become effective in two weeks which would be within the next two days.

Miss Rowe turned to Miss Mann at this point and said: "I guess I spoke too soon a week ago when I told you we had plenty of staff."

MISS MANN: You can't predict from one week to the next. Miss Connor hasn't been with you long, has she?

MISS ROWE: She began sometime last fall. We don't have any staff nurse on the service who has been with us for over a year and a half.

The conference between the two supervisors ended in a few minutes, and each went to her respective service to make rounds. Miss Mann accompanied Miss Rowe to her wards.

Upon arriving on Ward 5, Miss Rowe was approached by Miss Connor. She nodded a greeting in Miss Mann's direction before she spoke to Miss Rowe.

MISS CONNOR: Do you have a minute, Miss Rowe, I would like to speak with you?

MISS ROWE: Yes, I have.

Miss Rowe remained standing at one side of the corridor. Miss Connor looked toward the solarium as a likely place to go to talk, but Miss Rowe did not take the hint, so Miss Connor continued: "You have

* Permission was granted by the Board of Trustees of Boston University to reprint this case contained in *Case Studies in Nursing Service Administration,* Volume II, compiled by the faculty and graduate students of Boston University School of Nursing, and copyrighted 1954 by the Board of Trustees of Boston University. Copies of the case may be obtained through the Boston University Book Store (31/SBMMCR).

perhaps already learned that I handed in my resignation two weeks ago for this coming Friday. I have found the commuting distance too great and the hours so irregular that it is difficult to find enough time for study. I have decided to transfer to —— Hospital which will be a lot more convenient for me."

MISS ROWE: Yes, I was informed that you had resigned while I was on vacation. I am very sorry to have you leave us, but I can see your point of view. I hope you will enjoy your work at —— Hospital.

MISS CONNOR: I don't know whether Miss James has given you the overtime slip for last week, but I am owed three hours. I would appreciate having that time made up to me this Friday, instead of receiving the extra pay. If I can get off at 1:00 P.M., I can get a ride to my home which will be a considerable saving in time and money for me. I intend to spend next week at home since it is spring vacation at the university.

MISS ROWE: I haven't seen the slips yet, but I will check over Friday's time sheet with Miss James, and we will try and arrange your time for you.

MISS CONNOR: Thank you very much.

When Miss Rowe finished checking on patients' conditions, she looked at the weekly time sheet and spoke with Miss James about giving Miss Connor her three hours of make-up time. They agreed they could give it to her on Friday, so Miss Rowe asked Miss James to inform her. Miss Rowe did not confer with Miss Connor again before she terminated her employment.

As Miss Mann thought over Miss Connor's conversation with Miss Rowe, she wondered what other reasons Miss Connor had for wanting a change in position. Her excuses about having to spend so much time commuting and the frequent split hours were significant factors, but not major enough to cause her to resign, providing she was stimulated in her job and deriving satisfaction from it. Miss Mann decided she would try and arrange to have coffee with her Friday morning and see what she could find out.

Miss Mann had had an opportunity during her observations on the pediatric unit over a period of several months to chat with Miss Connor on numerous occasions. She was a quiet, serious girl, who was very conscientious and detailed in her work. She appeared to enjoy her patients. She approached all the children with a calm, even-tempered manner and had little difficulty gaining their cooperation.

Miss Connor did not socialize to any extent with many of the staff; she often went to morning coffee alone. She was not unfriendly, however, and was always eager to chat when approached. She had recently graduated from a collegiate nursing school and was now working toward a master's degree in education.

Friday morning when Miss Mann arrived at the hospital, she went directly to Miss Connor's ward and looked her up. She was in the midst of bathing Sue, one of her patients, when Miss Mann stuck her head around the curtain.

Miss Mann: Good morning, Miss Connor. Good morning, Sue. How are you this morning?

Sue: Fine. I can get up this morning and I was just operated upon yesterday!

Miss Mann: Isn't that wonderful that you feel so well! (Pause) Miss Connor—I would like to join you for coffee when you go down. Would you look me up? I'll be around on the ward.

Miss Connor: Fine, Miss Mann, I will be free in about a half hour.

Miss Connor joined Miss Mann in about forty-five minutes and they left for coffee. On their way to the cafeteria they chatted amiably about Miss Connor's vacation, her home, and where it was located. Once they were seated at the table with their coffee, Miss Connor turned toward Miss Mann and spoke seriously.

Miss Connor: I think you are aware that Miss Rowe and I have not hit it off from the very start. I found her cold and impersonal. She doesn't take an interest in any of us. I am not the only one who feels this way. That is what you wanted to know, isn't it?

Miss Mann (smiling): I am interested in what you say, because up until this point I could only surmise these relationships from my observations. No one who is still working in the situation is going to feel free to be so frank.

Miss Connor: You receive no recognition for having a brain around here. When the head nurse or assistant head nurse is off duty on split time, there is always a nursing student from their own school left in charge over the graduate nurse. That would be fine if it was to give the student administrative experience, but they act as if we were not capable. We never get a report; doctors come up to you with questions assuming you are in charge, and you feel like a fool because you don't know the answers. Information about the patients is never passed along so you can learn anything. There is so little time on day duty to read charts. I did get to one of those psychiatric conferences, but it was only because the doctor invited me, as I had been interested in knowing how to handle Donny better and had spoken to this psychiatrist several times when he was on the ward. When I returned, I gave Miss James a complete report of the conference, but that is as far as it went.

MISS MANN: That is the only staff education opportunity you feel you have had?

MISS CONNOR: Yes, there is no general program and nothing within the department, except for brief, superficial conferences following morning report occasionally. I have never had a chance to attend doctors' rounds.

MISS MANN: Another thing I am interested in is your opinion of your orientation period, if you can remember back four or five months.

MISS CONNOR (with a short laugh): What orientation! Oh, Miss Hood was very nice to me, but she isn't responsible for all the information you need to know before you can work effectively on pediatrics. All of that I learned by myself the hard way. You remember that farce of a conference Miss Rowe had with the three of us staff nurses, because she wanted to shift us to different floors before there was a complete change of students. It would give us time to adjust and make less confusion during the student change! She never changed both groups at the same time! Only I got changed two weeks later, the same day as the students. The week before that, after working here only two weeks I was put on nights because the rotation plan for the students got fouled up just before they were to finish their affiliation. Oh, I could go on and on—!

MISS MANN: I am grateful for this opportunity to talk with you. Are you all set to begin your new job when you come back from vacation?

MISS CONNOR: Yes, I was greeted with open arms. There is a new floor that has been opened on surgery, and the director offered me the assistant head nurse position which had not been filled.

MISS MANN: Isn't that wonderful! It isn't pediatrics, I take it?

MISS CONNOR: No. I hadn't made up my mind which I preferred, children or adults, so I thought I would try pediatrics here, but I think I would just as soon have adult surgery. I'll see how things work out.

MISS MANN: Well, thank you for your help and good luck to you. We better be heading back to the floor.

ASSIGNMENT TO GROUP DISCUSSANTS

How can Miss Rowe, supervisor, identify how subordinates perceive their relationships with her?

Are Miss Connor's private reasons for resigning unique, or may they be causes of dissatisfactions in others?

What needs to be done to prevent other resignations?

Hampton Hospital *

Hampton Hospital, a large general hospital, is located in a metropolitan area and draws its employees from the city in which it is situated and from the surrounding suburbs as well. The nursing service department employs graduate staff nurses, trained nursing aides, and clerical workers on its various units. Students from the school of nursing conducted by the hospital and from several affiliated institutions obtain their clinical experience on the ward and private floors of the institution.

This hospital, like the majority of hospitals today, provides a midmorning coffee hour in its cafeteria—the coffee hour appears at times to be the counterpart of the old New England cracker barrel session.

One morning, during the coffee hour, Madeline Hayes, the medical supervisor, was discussing the problem of tardiness among the personnel with a group of supervisors.

MADELINE: It seems to me that the attitude of people toward their work has changed. The head nurses don't get on duty on time in the morning and they're behind all day—the students are late—and the lay personnel, later. Believe me, when I was a head nurse, I was on my floor at ten minutes of seven, took the report, and got things started.

HELEN PHILBRICK (supervisor of the private pavilion): It's all in the way you're brought up. Our superintendent of nurses never excused tardiness. You couldn't be late in giving a treatment or a medicine, let alone coming on duty late. There was no use in giving her an excuse because she didn't recognize one. Nowadays, if you accept a good excuse, you set a precedent and don't know where to stop.

ROSE ZELL (supervisor): Well, that was in the old days. The graduates lived in the nurses' homes, and there weren't the numbers of aides and orderlies that we have today. A lot of nurses have to get youngsters ready for school and pack lunches before they start off in

* Permission was granted by the Board of Trustees of Boston University to modify and reprint this case from *Case Studies in Nursing Service Administration,* Volume I, compiled by the faculty and graduate students of Boston University School of Nursing, and copyrighted 1954 by the Board of Trustees of Boston University. Copies of the unmodified case may be obtained through the Boston University Book Store (11/MGHH9).

the morning; and I have one head nurse who uses three kinds of transportation to get here in the morning. If a bus schedule changes, as on Sundays or holidays, she's thrown off schedule.

MARY RITCHIE (obstetrical supervisor): I think the lay personnel are the greatest offenders.

HELEN: Oh, I don't know about that. The idea that head nurses should be on duty at ten minutes of seven in the morning has certainly gone by the board.* I have one head nurse who gets on duty at 6:30, but she's a rarity. The others pretty much try to hit seven o'clock, but I don't think they consider five or ten minutes after seven as being late. I'll wager that the only people who would be called late here are the ones who appear on duty a half hour late day after day.

MARGARET SHEAFFER (a late arriver): I don't know what you're discussing, but if it's about getting to work on time, I sure have gastric ulcers today—being Friday.† But if I'm five minutes late on Tuesday, Thursday, or Saturday, I don't get into a dither over it. I don't know that my conscience would smite me too hard until I was ten minutes late.

ROSE MARIE CLEARY (supervisor): Gee, I know how you feel. The first week I was back after vacation, I couldn't seem to get back on schedule. I was late for the supervisors' conference on Monday; then I couldn't get the car started on Wednesday, so I was late again. By Friday, I felt so guilty I felt like making a public apology, because I got tangled up in the traffic and was late again.

MADELINE: Well, I'll be travelling along. See you at the meeting.

As Madeline Hayes walked out of the dining-room, Jean Crowley, a head nurse on one of the medical wards seated at an adjoining table, turned to her friend, Ruth Elwell, and said: "I never eat breakfast, you know, but yesterday around 8:30, I just had to come down here to get something to eat. The supervisors certainly eyed me for being off the ward. I notice that some of *them* manage to eat *their* breakfast after they report on duty."

RUTH: What time do the supervisors work anyway? I've never known.

JEAN: Well, I guess they work 7:30 to 4:00, but I don't know that I was ever told. I sort of surmised it, as I did when they stopped working split time.

---

* It was a policy of the hospital that head nurses be on duty at 6:50 A.M.
† Supervisors' conferences with the Director of Nursing Service were held every Monday, Wednesday, and Friday at 7:30 A.M.

EVELYN COX (head nurse): What are you two so grumpy about this morning? (As she appeared with a cup of coffee and a doughnut and pulled up a chair next to Jean.)

JEAN: I just got off to a bad start this morning. Had to call down a couple of kids this morning for coming on late and, on top of that, my aide didn't show up until nine, and she was supposed to come on at seven. These students don't get enough sleep—they have too many late leaves and overnights, and then they can't get up in the morning.

EVELYN: What about your aide—too many late leaves too?

JEAN: Your guess is as good as mine. The time slip has been right there on the desk all week, but she says that she thought that she was supposed to work nine to five today. How can you tell if she really did make a mistake or overslept and is making out that she was mistaken? Anyway, she's a good worker when she does get here. I don't know how I'd get along without her.

EVELYN: Last Saturday, my ward clerk did the same thing. First, she forgot what day it was, and then she forgot that the bus schedule was different on Saturdays.

Jean and Ruth returned to their floors, leaving Evelyn to finish her coffee. Norma Greene, the assistant head nurse on the maternity floor, came up to the table.

NORMA: Why didn't you wait for me?

EVELYN: I went down and waited for fifteen minutes, but you were busy. Then Miss Ritchie came along and asked me if I had any errands to do before going to coffee because you would be tied up for awhile. So I went along to the pharmacy—

NORMA: Busy on your floor today?

EVELYN: Not too bad, but busy enough.

NORMA: I wish we could say that. This being paid overtime is fine, but when you have to work overtime every single day, it gets pretty tiresome.

EVELYN: Why don't you get your work organized?

NORMA: Organized! I don't know how you can organize when two and three patients land back from the recovery room at three o'clock and all the students go off to class. I feel that I have to stay on, but I don't feel that anyone knows I'm there or why I'm there. Sure, I'd like to go off on time, but—

EVELYN: Well, I know how it is, but at least on our floor, we seem to be catching up a little these past couple of weeks. Before, we were just about an hour behind all day long.

NORMA: What's the secret?

EVELYN: The night nurses only wash the very sick patients and take the temps in the morning, so they're ready to give the report by five after seven. Before, we were standing around until fifteen or twenty minutes past seven waiting for them to finish up.

NORMA: I should think it would take as much time to wash the rest of the patients.

EVELYN: The aides do that during the report. Then they get a report on their own patients afterward. They don't take in the report anyway —too complicated.

BARBARA MOORE (head nurse, joining them): Morning reports—one minute after they're over, no one knows a thing that's been said. Ask anyone a question about a patient, and no one can answer. If anyone does remember, it's because they've scribbled something down on a scrap of paper.

RACHEL TOLMAN (a newcomer to the table): Who's talking about morning reports?

EVELYN: I guess you and Barbara will have to settle it. Norma and I have to be on our way.

RACHEL: Believe me, I'm going to have my morning report at seven o'clock. Anyone who wants to hear it had better be there. My assistant showed up ten minutes late this morning, and I'm not going to wait for her again. The report is going to be given at seven and let the night people off duty. I worked on a floor here where the head nurse puttered around fifteen or twenty minutes every morning waiting for people to show up on duty, and I'm not going to do the same thing, although (she laughed) I was usually the late one. Figured I might as well stay in bed as wait around for her to get started.

A week later, the question of tardiness came up at the supervisors' conference in connection with the method of handling supervisory problems in general.

MISS MORAN (assistant director of nursing): Don't you think that the tardiness is a definite problem in this institution?

MADELINE HAYES: I think it's more than a problem of tardiness— it's almost a general attitude of indifference toward punctuality. But a supervisor is a little hesitant to speak about tardiness because she may not know how late the nurses or students worked the day before. I know that I have no way of knowing unless I make a special trip to the nursing office to find out. As a supervisor, I feel that I ought to commend a student or a graduate on her good attendance record, but the way it turns out, I'm usually only conscious of those who are chronic offenders at being late.

ROSE ZELL: Now, I have one head nurse who is always on time, but you'd know that to look at her. She's immaculately neat about herself, and everything at the desk is always in its place. But one of my other head nurses, who does really a fine job, just can't seem to get herself here on time in the morning. I know that she tries, but I can't figure it out. Maybe I ought to be more authoritarian. The funny thing about it is that she worked as a staff nurse before taking this head nurse job and was always on time. Basically, I think tardiness is resistance to something.

AMY DAHL (supervisor of the nursing aides): I think people get bored sometimes and don't realize what ails them. I have moved a few people who were chronically tardy on one unit and found that they were always on time on the new unit. I think it makes a difference whether or not a person feels that she has to relieve the night people too. Of course, the problem with lay personnel seems to be absenteeism rather than tardiness. But, if they are late, they don't seem to want to make the time up. I really think they'd rather lose the pay.

ROSE ZELL: Do the rest of you find that the nurses on your units write down 7 to 3:30 on the time sheet regardless of what time they arrive on duty?

Most of the supervisors nodded in agreement, but one spoke up to say: "I can't say that it's only the day people that are late. The relief people are just the same. They feel that their work begins when the day people go off, I guess."

MISS MORAN (interrupting): I don't know that we have arrived at any conclusions but our time is drawing to a close.

As the group arose to leave the conference, Nora Meyers, one of the out-patient department supervisors who had hurried out ahead of the others, was heard saying as she passed through the door: "—the answer is time clocks. Anyone who wants to get to work on time can do it if they want to. All this business about resist—" and her voice trailed off in the distance.

Miss Moran looked up at the remaining supervisors with a smile and said, "Do you think Miss Meyers might be right—that people can get to work on time if they really want to?"

MADELINE HAYES: It may be more than that—it may be a matter of moral obligation.

MISS MORAN: Why don't you think this thing through and next week let us see if we can identify the basic problem and determine what should be done about it?

ASSIGNMENT TO GROUP DISCUSSANTS

Are tardiness and absenteeism always symptoms of resistance? What is the range of possible underlying factors?

Reprimand, punishment, time clocks—do these affect change toward improvement? What different approaches are possible?

How do the attitudes of the head nurses and supervisors contribute to the tardiness problem?

Mrs. Brown, Head Nurse *

It was 8:30 A.M., Friday, as Miss Reed, medical-surgical supervisor, made her way down the corridor of Ward A.† She passed Mrs. Brown, the head nurse, and heard her say to Miss Smith,‡ "Will you take over the team leadership for South? Mrs. Cross § is not coming in."

Miss Reed was startled to hear Miss Smith retort in what seemed a sharp and angry tone, "No, I won't. I'm sick and tired of being considered good enough to be a team leader when no R.N. is available and then being yanked off the job when one is. Also I'm tired of being moved back and forth from East to South."

Miss Reed went on her way without stopping but planned to check with Mrs. Brown before she left the ward. Her rounds over, Miss Reed approached the desk in time to overhear Mrs. Brown saying to the ward clerk,‖ "I don't know what I'm going to do with Miss Smith. All she gives me is sass. Today she wouldn't even do what I asked her to. She's getting too big for her boots."

Miss Reed observed that the ward clerk made no reply to this comment. She had observed that two students and a doctor were in a position to overhear the comment, too. Miss Reed then drew Mrs. Brown aside to ask if they might arrange for a conference to discuss ward problems. A time was set.

Mrs. Brown came into the conference room with what seemed a grim expression on her face. She dropped into the easy chair, drew out a cigarette, and sighed. Miss Reed began. "Because I know it is difficult to manage when we are short of regular full-time help, I

---

* Permission to modify and reprint this case was granted by Mrs. Winifred Griffin, R.N., Associate Director for Regional Nursing Programs, New England Board of Higher Education, and Nurse Consultant to the New England Council on Higher Education for Nursing. The assignment to group discussants is that of the authors.
† Ward A is a 24-bed nonsegregated adult medical-surgical service. It is divided into two wings, East and South. South is in an older building and is considered to have less desirable accommodations.
‡ An L.P.N. (licensed practical nurse) who works full time.
§ An R.N. (registered professional nurse) who works regularly three days a week.
‖ A former L.P.N. who because of physical limitations has become a ward clerk.

wondered how you were making out. I couldn't help overhearing Miss Smith's remark this morning. I wondered what was behind the difficulty and how you handled it."

Mrs. Brown bit her lips and said, "Well, you know how it is. The same old problem—not enough people and too much to do. These part-timers with 'can't get in' make me sick. The patients still have to be cared for. Look at today—I had fixed it so Mrs. Cross and Mrs. Grant * could be team leaders on South since Mrs. Cross was working 7 to 12 noon and Mrs. Grant was on 11:30 to 3:30 P.M. I had put an aide and a student on with them. I had put Mrs. Lee † as team leader on East and given her Miss Smith and a student. So when I get the message about Mrs. Cross not coming in, I asked Miss Smith to be team leader and she says 'No.' I'm so tired of fighting with Smith that I didn't force the issue. Instead I turned over to Mary ‡ the making out of the dietary and admission and discharge list, and the transferring of new orders, and acted as team leader myself."

Miss Reed: How did it go?

Mrs. Brown: Well, I sure was busy and we didn't get a stat order of mercuhydrine given on time. That didn't matter too much since we had to wait on the pharmacy to send it up, but I'm getting real fed-up with this job. It's not worth the little extra pay to take such a beating.

Miss Reed: You're taking a beating?

Mrs. Brown: Yes, I am. Everyone seems out to get me. They talk about me behind my back, correct me in front of others, refuse to do what I want done, and even tell lies about me. Why do you know that yesterday Miss Ford § called me at home to say that Miss Smith told her that I'd forgotten to get a written order for an enema from Doctor Roberts? ‖ What right has she got to say that? Doctor Roberts has told me that anytime I think the patient needs an enema to see that it is given. Then take Thursday. I was checking a post-op's i.v. It had gone into the tissues. I started to remove it when Miss Vell #

---

* Mrs. Cross and Mrs. Grant are registered nurses who work somewhat irregularly on a part-time basis.
† Mrs. Lee is a regular full-time registered nurse.
‡ The ward clerk.
§ A part-time registered nurse who was a social acquaintance of Mrs. Brown.
‖ One of the older staff men who had been associated with the hospital for many years.
A nursing aide who had had two years in a diploma program.

came in. She said she was sure it was running O.K. since everytime she'd pinched the tube, she'd gotten back blood. She'd pinched the tube! What right does she have to do that? Boy, was I mad. I held my temper until I got her into the utility room and then did I give her a blast. But the last straw was yesterday when I spoke to a student about a greasy ring in the patient's washbasin. The student said that she had been so busy with her two pre-op patients and her C.V.A. that she had just used a paper towel to wipe it out. The student had the nerve to ask me what was more important—the patients or the housekeeping. Aside from her being rude, I think a good nurse should be able to get everything done.

Miss Reed listened with interest to the comments. She had already heard about the aide's version of the i.v. problem. Coming on duty Wednesday morning, she had found a note on her desk saying that the aide intended to resign. She had arranged a conference with her during which Miss Vell had cried about the brutal "call-down" she had been given.

Miss Vell had given this version of the "call-down": "I've had two years of nurse's training. We were taught how to check an i.v. for infiltration and were expected to do it. I don't see why Mrs. Brown gets so upset about a small thing like that when she asks me to do other things like irrigating a Foley catheter which I have never been taught."

As the conference with Miss Vell continued, Miss Reed found out that Miss Vell was aware of what the hospital expected of its aides and also that a list of permitted duties was posted on the ward bulletin board for nursing personnel. She also got the impression that when help was short, the limits of the list were overlooked. When she had asked Miss Vell why she had not told Mrs. Brown how she felt, Miss Vell replied, "You can't talk to her. Even when we had ward conferences, no one ever spoke up. Mrs. Brown does all the talking."

Miss Reed had also learned about the apparent emphasis on housekeeping on Ward A at the supervisor meeting with the educational personnel.

Having this information, Miss Reed suggested that perhaps it would be helpful if Mrs. Brown and she studied the nursing needs on the unit to see if a different staffing pattern would help. She did not, however, hold out hope of finding any more full-time registered nurses. She suggested that in preparation for this conference Mrs. Brown might have Mary collect on a prepared form certain information about the nursing needs of the patients—the types and number of the supportive and therapeutic treatments carried out, as well as the degree of dependency of the patients. She also asked whether Mrs. Brown had been holding the weekly staff meetings. She learned that they had been omitted for three weeks because of a shortage of personnel and because Mrs. Brown did not really feel comfortable about conducting these meetings. She suggested that Mrs. Brown schedule one in the near future to "clear the air," and at Mrs. Brown's suggestion she agreed to attend as an observer. She also suggested that the part-timers be invited to attend. As Mrs. Brown left, she gave her a simple booklet describing ways of conducting such a conference.

ASSIGNMENT TO GROUP DISCUSSANTS

What would be your "supervisory diagnosis"?

What supervisory plan would you formulate to assist Mrs. Brown?

What plan of action would you institute to achieve the objectives of your plan?

Situation I *

The head nurse put the phone back on the hook. "Set up 102 for diabetic in coma. Mr. Krosick is back again." "What," said the nurse, "we sent him home well controlled last week. I wonder what went wrong." Subsequently, they both learned that Mr. Krosick, a construction worker with an out-of-state pipeline company, had not stayed on his diet or taken insulin by test. He had been joining the boys at the corner beer parlor for the usual beer on his way home from work. This had been his usual custom, and he saw no reason to change. In addition, he hadn't wanted to test his urine before his noon lunch because all the men carried lunch pails and sat down in the fields together. So he'd been approximating what he needed and added this to his morning dose of insulin.

ASSIGNMENT TO GROUP DISCUSSANTS

Divide group into two sections. Ask one to assume the role of the head nurse; the other, the role of the supervisor. Work collaboratively on a nursing care plan which would include patient teaching. Then plan how to involve all personnel in implementing this plan for Mr. Krosick.

Situation II *

The head nurse noted the repetitive buzz and flash of the signal light 201, as she went into the treatment room. Two minutes later it was still sounding when she came back to the station. "Oh, is the bell stuck again?" she said. The ward clerk, drawing her body in tightly, narrowing her lips, glared, "No, it's just Mr. Lord again. He's really getting to be a pest, always wanting the nurse, never needing her. I'm getting so I just ignore him, and so do the others."

The head nurse, from previous experience recognized the ward clerk's behavior as frustration, nodded, and started down the corridor.

* Permission to modify and reprint this situation was granted by Mrs. Winifred Griffin, R.N., Associate Director for Regional Nursing Programs, New England Board of Higher Education, and Nurse Consultant to the New England Council on Higher Education for Nursing. The assignment to group discussants is that of the authors.

"How on earth am I going to help my staff work with difficult, demoralizing patients?" Entering Mr. Lord's room, she asked if she could help him. "I want to get over on my side; my leg hurts," he said. Then, as she positioned him, he continued, "The nurses ignore me. They don't like me. No one cares if I hurt or not." Only inwardly did the head nurse agree, saying to herself, "How true. What do I really want my people to know in order that they can work with people like Mr. Lord?"

ASSIGNMENT TO GROUP DISCUSSANTS

Assume the role of the head nurse. How would you bring about a change of attitude in the ward secretary toward such a patient as Mr. Lord? Assuming that the head nurse may have observed need for change of attitudes in other categories of workers, how would she modify her plan for them?

Variation of the Case Method

In order to expand the experience of developing skills and collaborative problem-solving and decision-making, we are including four assignments. They may stimulate the members to use the seminar for the systematic examination of their own situations.

CONFLICT

Describe a conflict situation in which you are or have been personally involved. What are some of the factors contributing to the problem? What has led up to the conflict? What are the positions of other people involved in this situation?

What are the available resources or aids that might assist you in remedying this problem?

1. Which of these resources or aids are of major importance?
2. Which are of moderate value?
3. Which are of minimum value?

NEGATIVE CRITICAL INCIDENT

Looking back over your experience in your department, think of an event that occurred in which you played a prominent and effective part and in which the outcome was unfavorable. Suggestions for analysis are as follows:

To whom was the outcome unfavorable?

Self
Patient (s)
Technical-Personal
System
Others

Who initiated the action?

Nurse
Subordinate
Peer
Superiors

Was the situation predominantly?

Interpersonnel
Patient Care
Teaching
Mixed
Administrative
Organizational
Maintenance
Other

Was the problem a hierarchical or nonhierarchical one? If hierarchical, did it involve subordinates or superiors? Was there conflict caused by differences in role perception, or role expectation?

Specification of the conditions leading up to the action.

TODAY'S DILEMMA

Describe a problem of supervision that you are struggling with now.

When a problem occurs, we usually think of certain *pressures* that have been instrumental in creating this problem, and of certain *resources* that might be used to remedy it. List the relevant pressures and resources in your situation.

What action do you think should be taken in order to remedy your situation?

Should there be a long-range plan of action as well as short-range decisions?

INTERPERSONAL INCIDENT

1. Describe briefly the incident that occurred (who was involved, what happened).

2. What did you do and say at the time?

3. How did you feel during the incident (rank order)?

_____angry   _____defensive   _____frustrated
_____pleased   _____helpful   _____helpless
_____indifferent _____uncertain

4. What do you think caused the incident?

5. Were these causes based on facts, feelings, or inference?

6. Did you check your perceptions of the incident or its causes with others? If so, were you looking for confirmation of your own views?

7. Did you blame others? Do you still?

8. Was it within your power to change the situation?

9. Would you handle the situation differently now?

SELECTED BIBLIOGRAPHY

The following is a list of books we believe will be relevant and helpful to use in connection with the cases and the sections on the philosophy of dynamic supervision and adult education. We believe, however, that the focus of in-service training in the supervisory process should be more on the analysis of cases, rather than on reading assignments.

Abdellah, Faye, *et al. Patient-Centered Approaches to Nursing*. New York: The Macmillan Company, 1960.

American Nurses' Association. *Standards for Organized Nursing Services*. New York: American Nurses' Association, 1965.

Argyris, Chris. *Interpersonal Competence and Organizational Effectiveness*. Homewood, Ill.: Dorsey Press, 1962.

Barrett, Jean. *The Head Nurse*. New York: Appleton-Century-Crofts, 1962.

Bradford, Leland P.; Gibb, Jack L.; and Benne, Kenneth D. (eds.). *T-Group Theory and Laboratory Method: Innovation in Re-Education*. New York: John Wiley & Sons, 1964.

Brown, David S. *The Leader Looks at Decision Making*. Monograph #6. Washington: Leadership Resources, Inc., 1961.

Brown, Esther Lucille. *Newer Dimensions of Patient Care*, Part I. New York: Russell Sage Foundation, 1961.

————. *Newer Dimensions of Patient Care*, Part II. New York: Russell Sage Foundation, 1962.

Gibb, Jack, *et al. Dynamics of Participative Groups*. St. Louis: John S. Swift Company, 1951.

Haire, Mason (ed.). *Modern Organization Theory.* New York: John Wiley & Sons, 1960.

Kidd, J. Roby. *How Adults Learn.* New York: Association Press, 1959.

Knowles, Malcolm, and Knowles, Hulda. *How to Develop Better Leaders.* New York: Association Press, 1955.

———. *Introduction to Group Dynamics.* New York: Association Press, 1959.

Kron, Thora. *Nursing Team Leadership.* Philadelphia: W. B. Saunders Company, 1961.

Lippett, Gorden L. *The Leader Looks at Group Effectiveness.* Monograph #3. Washington: Leadership Resources, Inc., 1961.

MacGregor, Frances Cooke. *Social Science in Nursing.* New York: Russell Sage Foundation, 1960.

Maier, Norman R. F. *Problem-Solving Discussions and Conferences: Leadership Methods and Skills.* New York: McGraw-Hill Book Company, 1963.

———. *Supervisory and Executive Development.* New York: John Wiley & Sons, 1960.

Mauksch, Hans O., and Tagliacozzo, Daisy L. *The Patient's View of the Patient Role.* Part I, "Analysis of Interviews." Chicago: Department of Patient Care Research, Presbyterian–St. Luke's Hospital, 1962. Reprints available from IIT Health Research Center, Illinois Institute of Technology, Chicago, Ill.

McNair, Malcolm (ed.). *The Case Method at Harvard Business School.* New York: McGraw-Hill Book Company, Inc., 1954.

Meyer, Genevieve. *Tenderness and Technique.* Los Angeles: Institute of Industrial Relations, University of California, 1960.

Miles, Matthew B. *Learning to Work in Groups.* New York: Columbia University Press, 1959.

National League for Nursing, Department of Hospital Nursing. *Blueprint for Action in Hospital Nursing.* New York: National League for Nursing, 1964.

———. *Criteria for Evaluating a Hospital Department of Nursing Service.* New York: National League for Nursing, 1965.

———. *In Pursuit of Quality: Hospital Nursing Services.* New York: National League for Nursing, 1964.

National Training Laboratories. *Leadership in Action.* Selected Reading Series 1. Washington: National Education Association, 1961.

Perrodin, Cecelia. *Supervision of Nursing Personnel*. New York: The Macmillan Company, 1954.

Schein, Edgar H., and Bennis, Warren G. *Personal and Organizational Change Through Group Methods*. New York: John Wiley & Sons, 1965.

Tannenbaum, Robert, and Schmidt, Warren H. "How to Choose a Leadership Pattern," *Harvard Business Review*, XXXVI (March–April, 1958), pp. 95–101.

Tannenbaum, Robert; Weschler, Irving; and Massarik, Fred. *Leadership and Organization: A Behavioral Science Approach*. New York: McGraw-Hill Book Company, 1961.

U.S. Department of Health, Education, and Welfare, Public Health Service, Division of Nursing. *How to Study Nursing Activities in a Patient Unit*. Washington: U.S. Government Printing Office, 1964.